Laparoscopic Approaches in Oncology

Editor

JAMES FLESHMAN

SURGICAL ONCOLOGY CLINICS OF NORTH AMERICA

www.surgonc.theclinics.com

Consulting Editor
NICHOLAS J. PETRELLI

January 2013 • Volume 22 • Number 1

ELSEVIER

1600 John F. Kennedy Boulevard • Suite 1800 • Philadelphia, PA 19103-2899

http://www.theclinics.com

SURGICAL ONCOLOGY CLINICS OF NORTH AMERICA Volume 22, Number 1
January 2013 ISSN 1055-3207, ISBN-13: 978-1-4557-4950-8

Editor: Jessica McCool

Surgical Oncology Clinics of North America (ISSN 1055-3207) is published quarterly by Elsevier Inc., 360 Park Avenue South, New York, NY 10010-1710. Months of publication are January, April, July, and October. Business and Editorial Offices: 1600 John F. Kennedy Blvd., Ste. 1800, Philadelphia, PA 19103-2899. Customer Service Office: 3251 Riverport Lane, Maryland Heights, MO 63043. Periodicals postage paid at New York, NY and additional mailing offices. Subscription prices are $274.00 per year (US individuals), $401.00 (US institutions) $135.00 (US student/resident), $314.00 (Canadian individuals), $498.00 (Canadian institutions), $193.00 (Canadian student/resident), $392.00 (foreign individuals), $498.00 (foreign institutions), and $193.00 (foreign student/resident). Foreign air speed delivery is included in all *Clinics* subscription prices. All prices are subject to change without notice. **POSTMASTER**: Send address changes to *Surgical Oncology Clinics of North America,* Elsevier Health Science Division, Subscription Customer Service, 3251 Riverport Lane, Maryland Heights, MO 63043. **Customer Service: 1-800-654-2452 (US and Canada). 314-447-8871 (outside U.S. and Canada). Fax: 314-447-8029. E-mail: journalscustomerservice-usa@elsevier.com** (for print support); **journalsonline support-usa@elsevier.com** (for online support).

Reprints. For copies of 100 or more, of articles in this publication, please contact the Commercial Reprints Department, Elsevier Inc., 360 Park Avenue South, New York, New York 10010-1710. Tel. 212-633-3813; Fax: 212-462-1935; E-mail: reprints@elsevier.com.

Surgical Oncology Clinics of North America is covered in *MEDLINE/PubMed (Index Medicus)* and *EMBASE/ Excerpta Medica, Current Contents/Clinical Medicine, and ISI/BIOMED.*

Printed and bound by CPI Group (UK) Ltd, Croydon, CR0 4YY

Transferred to digital print 2012

Contributors

CONSULTING EDITOR

NICHOLAS J. PETRELLI, MD
Bank of America Endowed Medical Director, Helen F. Graham Cancer Center at Christiana Care Health System, Newark, Delaware

GUEST EDITOR

JAMES FLESHMAN, MD
Professor of Surgery, Washington University School of Medicine, St Louis, Missouri

AUTHORS

GERALD L. ANDRIOLE, MD
Division of Urologic Surgery, Washington University School of Medicine, St Louis, Missouri

SAM B. BHAYANI, MD
Division of Urologic Surgery, Washington University School of Medicine, St Louis, Missouri

JENNIFER CREAMER, MD
Department of General Surgery, William Beaumont Army Medical Center, El Paso, Texas

R. SHERBURNE FIGENSHAU, MD
Division of Urologic Surgery, Washington University School of Medicine, St Louis, Missouri

MICHEL GAGNER, MD, FACS
Minimally Invasive Surgery Section, Clinique Michel Gagner, Inc., Montreal, Quebec, Canada

WILLIAM E. GILLANDERS, MD
Professor, Department of Surgery, Washington University School of Medicine, St Louis, Missouri

WILLIAM G. HAWKINS, MD, FACS
Associate Professor of Surgery, Section of Hepatobiliary, Pancreatic and Gastrointestinal Surgery, Department of Surgery, Washington University School of Medicine, St Louis, Missouri

DANIEL B. JONES, MD, MS, FACS
Department of Surgery, Beth Israel Deaconess Medical Center, Harvard Medical School, Boston, Massachusetts

OMAR YUSEF KUDSI, MD, MBA
Fellow in Surgery, Department of Surgery, Beth Israel Deaconess Medical Center, Harvard Medical School, Boston, Massachusetts

BRENT D. MATTHEWS, MD
Professor of Surgery and Chief, Section of Minimally Invasive Surgery, Department of Surgery, Washington University School of Medicine, St Louis, Missouri

BRYAN F. MEYERS, MD, MPH
Department of Surgery, Washington University School of Medicine, St Louis, Missouri

JONATHAN B. MITCHEM, MD
Resident Physician, Department of Surgery, Washington University School of Medicine, St Louis, Missouri

ALEXANDER P. NAGLE, MD
Associate Professor, Department of Surgery, Feinberg School of Medicine, Northwestern University, Chicago, Illinois

KENNETH G. NEPPLE, MD
Division of Urologic Surgery, Washington University School of Medicine, St Louis, Missouri

EDUARDO PARRA-DAVILA, MD, FACS, FASCRS
Director of Minimally Invasive and Colorectal Surgery, Director of Hernia and Abdominal Wall Reconstruction, Florida Hospital Celebration Health Campus, Celebration, Florida

JEFFREY H. PETERS, MD
Professor and Chair, Department of Surgery, University of Rochester School of Medicine and Dentistry, Rochester, New York

CHRISTIAN G. PEYRE, MD
Assistant Professor of Surgery, Department of Surgery, University of Rochester School of Medicine and Dentistry, Rochester, New York

JOSEPH D. PHILLIPS, MD
Department of Surgery, Feinberg School of Medicine, Northwestern University, Chicago, Illinois

VARUN PURI, MD
Department of Surgery, Washington University School of Medicine, St Louis, Missouri

SONIA RAMAMOORTHY, MD, FACS, FASCRS
Chief, Division of Colorectal Surgery; Associate Professor of Surgery, Rebecca and John Moores Cancer Center, University of California San Diego Health System, San Diego, California

GURDARSHAN S. SANDHU, MD
Division of Urologic Surgery, Washington University School of Medicine, St Louis, Missouri

NATHANIEL J. SOPER, MD
Loyal and Edith Davis Professor and Chair, Department of Surgery, Feinberg School of Medicine, Northwestern University, Chicago, Illinois

YOUSSEF S. TANAGHO, MD, MPH
Division of Urologic Surgery, Washington University School of Medicine, St Louis, Missouri

EMILY WINSLOW, MD
Assistant Professor of Surgery, Hepatopancreaticobiliary Surgery, Division of General Surgery, Department of Surgery, University of Wisconsin School of Medicine and Public Health, Madison, Wisconsin

Contents

This article focuses on endoscopic and robotic surgical techniques for the treatment of thyroid cancer. The most widely applied techniques are minimally invasive video-assisted thyroidectomy, as well as endoscopic techniques using a primarily axillary-based approach. Although there are few large studies delineating the benefits of endoscopic thyroid resection when compared with traditional thyroidectomy, in patients who desire the lack of a cervical incision, endoscopic thyroidectomy provides a safe and oncologically effective surgical option in the hands of experienced surgeons. Robotic surgical treatment of thyroid disease is a developing field and deserves further study before widespread application.

Minimally invasive surgery has revolutionized the surgical management of benign foregut disease, as well as pulmonary and other gastrointestinal malignancies. With the potential to reduce operative morbidity and increase patient satisfaction, minimally invasive esophagectomy for the management of esophageal cancer is gaining in popularity. It is unclear, however, whether the minimally invasive approach to esophageal cancer resection has comparable long-term oncologic results. This article discusses the rationale for minimally invasive esophagectomy, describes the surgical technique, and reviews the published results.

Surgical resection is currently the gold standard in operable patients with early-stage lung cancer. Video-assisted thoracoscopic surgery (VATS) lobectomy is a technique that has technically evolved and grown increasingly popular over the past two decades. This article presents the evolution, definition, current application, and some of the controversies surrounding VATS lobectomy.

Gastric cancer is common worldwide. Tumor location and disease stage differ between Asian and Western countries. Western patients often have higher BMIs and comorbidities that may make laparoscopic resections challenging. Multiple trials from Asian countries demonstrate the benefits of laparoscopic gastrectomy for early gastric cancer while maintaining equivalent short-term and long-term oncologic outcomes compared with open surgery. The outcomes of laparoscopy seem to offer equivalent results to open surgery. In the United States, laparoscopic gastrectomy remains in its infancy and is somewhat controversial. This article summarizes the literature on the epidemiology, operative considerations and approaches, and outcomes for laparoscopic gastrectomy.

The laparoscopic approach for benign and malignant lesions in the tail of the pancreas is becoming a more widely used approach. Multiple prospective studies have shown the feasibility and safety of laparoscopic distal pancreatectomy in single-center and multi-center settings. Laparoscopic distal pancreatectomy is a challenging procedure, because the pancreas is surrounded by critical structures and located in the retroperitoneum. Pancreatic fistula remains a common complication in the laparoscopic approach. Distal pancreatic aggressive tumors may not be appropriate for the laparoscopic approach due to the lack of oncologic safety studies.

Although most laparoscopic hepatic procedures are performed for benign disease, an increasing fraction is for malignant disease, including primary and metastatic liver tumors. Data suggest that minor and major hepatic resections are feasible and can be performed safely. The limited data currently available suggest that survival in patients with hepatocellular carcinoma and colorectal metastatic disease may be comparable to that achieved with open hepatectomy. The benefits of the laparoscopic approach seem to be shorter hospitalization, smaller incisions, and less blood loss. Despite the progress to date, concern continues about the potential for significant intraoperative hemorrhagic complications and oncologic outcomes.

This article provides an overview of extirpative laparoscopic and robotic procedures used in the management of renal cell carcinoma, including laparoscopic radical nephrectomy, laparoscopic partial nephrectomy, and robotic-assisted partial nephrectomy. The clinical indications and principles of surgical technique for each of these procedures are discussed. The oncologic, renal functional, and perioperative outcomes of these procedures are also assessed and compared, as are complication rates.

Laparoscopic procedures are preferred by surgeons and patients alike because of decreased pain, reduced perioperative morbidity, and an earlier return to self-reliance. During the last decade, laparoscopic adre-nalectomy has become the technique most commonly used for the removal of benign adrenal tumors. The indications for laparoscopy in malignant adrenal tumors remains controversial, because oncologic re-sections have not been reproducible compared with open techniques.

The purpose of this article is to provide an update on the current literature evaluating outcomes with laparoscopic prostatectomy. The reported peri-operative, oncologic, and functional outcomes with this approach are reviewed and comparisons are made to the open and robotic-assisted approaches.

Robotic approaches have seen significant growth in the last 5 years. Taking advantage of three-dimensional visualization, improved articulation, and multiple operating arms provides theoretical and real advantages in colorectal cancer surgery. This article reviews the potential advantages and disadvantages, current outcomes, and future directions for robotic approaches to colon cancer surgery.

SURGICAL ONCOLOGY
CLINICS OF NORTH AMERICA

Foreword

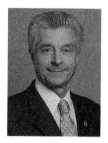

Nicholas J. Petrelli, MD
Consulting Editor

This issue of the *Surgical Oncology Clinics of North America* is entitled, "Laparoscopic Approaches in Oncology." The guest editor is James Fleshman, MD. Dr Fleshman is Professor of Surgery in the Division of General Surgery and Chief of the Section of Colon and Rectal Surgery at the Washington University School of Medicine. He is also Co-Director of the Gastrointestinal Center, Clinical Operations. Dr Fleshman completed his general surgery residency at the Jewish Hospital of St. Louis, and this was followed by a fellowship in colon and rectal surgery at the University of Toronto in Toronto, Canada. He is a member of the editorial board of *Diseases of Colon and Rectum*, the *Journal of Pelvic Surgery*, and the *Annals of Surgery*.

The last time the *Surgical Oncology Clinics of North America* put together an edition on laparoscopic surgery in oncology was July 2001. At that time, the consulting editor was Blake Cady, MD. Dr Cady stated in his foreword in 2001 that "the rush of emerging technology in surgery is no where more dramatically displayed than in the rapidly expanding use of endoscopic, laparoscopic and thoracoscopic instruments for diagnostic and therapeutic surgery." It would be fair to say 11 years later that "emerging technology in surgery" is now here and has been demonstrated by the outstanding group of authors that Dr Fleshman has organized in this edition of the *Surgical Oncology Clinics of North America*.

This edition of the *Surgical Oncology Clinics of North America* discusses the spectrum of laparoscopic approaches to cancers. The spectrum goes from minimally invasive surgery for esophageal cancer by Drs Peyre and Peters to laparoscopic prostatectomy by Dr Sandhu and associates and laparoscopic/robotic colectomy for colon cancer by Dr Davila and associates. The first laparoscopic procedure has been attributed to George Kelling, who was a surgeon from Dresden, although history relates that Dimitri Ott, a gynecologist from St. Petersburg, performed a laparoscopic procedure in the same year. Interestingly, Kelling introduced a cystoscope into a living dog through a small abdominal wall incision and examined the peritoneal cavity. To achieve a better view, a pneumoperitoneum was created by inserting a needle and injecting air filtered through sterile cotton. There is no question that we have come much further as demonstrated by Dr Fleshman and the outstanding group of authors he has put together for

Surg Oncol Clin N Am 22 (2013) ix–x
http://dx.doi.org/10.1016/j.soc.2012.08.011
1055-3207/13/$ – see front matter © 2013 Elsevier Inc. All rights reserved.

this issue of the *Surgical Oncology Clinics of North America*. The progress made in laparoscopic/robotic surgery has been amazing in the last 10 years and without question will continue to progress over the next decade.

I encourage senior surgeons to share the information in this issue of the *Surgical Oncology Clinics of North America* with their younger colleagues, surgical residents, and fellows.

Nicholas J. Petrelli, MD
Helen F. Graham Cancer Center
4701 Ogletown-Stanton Road, Suite 1213
Newark, DE 19713, USA

E-mail address:
npetrelli@christianacare.org

Preface

Laparoscopic Approaches in Oncology

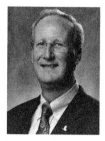

James Fleshman, MD
Guest Editor

As laparoscopy matures as a technique, we will be asking ourselves the question, "Is this technique appropriate for this cancer?" This issue was designed to provide insight into the current thought process of leaders in the area of oncology regarding the use of new approaches to their specific solid tumor of interest—specifically, laparoscopy and robotics. It may surprise some of us to see the controversy that remains in some areas of surgical oncology. I want to thank and congratulate the authors for their thorough and thoughtful contributions. It is my hope that we will look back in the next decade to this report and realize that all the issues and controversies have been resolved and surgical treatment of solid tumors with minimally invasive techniques is standard of care. Young surgical oncologists should take note, because careers can be founded on solving the problems highlighted in these articles.

James Fleshman, MD
Washington University School of Medicine
St Louis, MO, USA

E-mail address:
fleshman@wudosis.wustl.edu

Surg Oncol Clin N Am 22 (2013) xi
http://dx.doi.org/10.1016/j.soc.2012.08.008
1055-3207/13/$ – see front matter © 2013 Elsevier Inc. All rights reserved.

surgonc.theclinics.com

Endoscopic and Robotic Thyroidectomy for Cancer

Jonathan B. Mitchem, MD, William E. Gillanders, MD*

KEYWORDS

- Thyroid cancer • Robotic thyroidectomy • Endoscopic thyroidectomy

KEY POINTS

- Minimally invasive approaches for the surgical treatment of thyroid cancer are under investigation as a result of improvements in technology and the desire to avoid visible neck incisions.
- Multiple minimally invasive approaches to thyroid surgery have been used, including endoscopic thyroidectomy and robotic thyroidectomy. There is no clearly superior approach.
- Endoscopic and robotic thyroidectomy are still in the investigational phase, and further study is required to determine the appropriate context for the application of these techniques in the clinical setting.

INTRODUCTION

Thyroid cancer is the most common cancer of the endocrine system, and the fifth most common cancer affecting women in the United States, with approximately 56,000 expected new cases in 2012.[1] From 1999 to 2008, the incidence in thyroid cancer increased significantly, with the greatest increase noted in the diagnosis of localized disease, from 5.2 to 9.6 cases per 100,000 people.[2] This increase is largely believed to be related to improvements in diagnostic imaging, given that the largest increase has been observed in lesions less than 2.0 cm.[3] Most thyroid cancer is considered to be well-differentiated thyroid cancer (DTC), which includes papillary thyroid carcinoma (PTC), follicular thyroid carcinoma (FTC), and Hurthle cell carcinoma, with PTC comprising most of these cases. PTC and FTC have a favorable prognosis with 5-year survival of ~97% (http://www.cancer.gov/, 2012) and share recommendations regarding surgical therapy. Given that the greatest increase in thyroid cancer has been in patients with localized disease, the number of patients seeking surgical consultation for the treatment of thyroid cancer is expected to continue to increase.

Department of Surgery, Washington University School of Medicine, 660 South Euclid Avenue, St Louis, MO, USA
* Corresponding author.
E-mail address: gillandersw@wustl.edu

Surg Oncol Clin N Am 22 (2013) 1–13
http://dx.doi.org/10.1016/j.soc.2012.08.009
surgonc.theclinics.com
1055-3207/13/$ – see front matter

Recently, the American Thyroid Association (ATA) published revised evidence-based guidelines for the treatment of thyroid cancer, including surgical therapy.[4] Despite the acceptance of these guidelines by multiple endocrinology and endocrine surgery associations, controversies remain regarding optimal surgical therapy. The 2 main areas of controversy related to surgical therapy include the extent of thyroid resection (thyroid lobectomy vs total thyroidectomy) and the use of prophylactic central neck dissection (CND) in low-risk PTC, and papillary thyroid microcarcinoma (<10 mm, PTMC). It was recently shown in a large study of the American College of Surgeons National Cancer Data Base (more than 50,000 patients) that for PTC greater than 1 cm, total thyroidectomy decreased risk of recurrence and death when compared with those patients who underwent lobectomy; however, there was no difference in patients with PTC less than 1 cm.[5] A large study of the SEER (Surveillance Epidemiology and End Results) database from 1983 to 2002 showed no difference in 10-year overall survival or cancer-specific survival in patients undergoing thyroid lobectomy or total thyroidectomy for DTC,[6] although multivariate analysis suggested that total thyroidectomy was superior. Despite these results, controversy remains, because other studies have shown that tumor size has no effect on the incidence of contralateral disease,[7,8] and the clinical significance of contralateral disease is unclear.[9–11] The current ATA guidelines recommend that patients with a preoperative diagnosis of PTC greater than 1 cm undergo total or near-total thyroidectomy[4]; however, the appropriate surgical treatment of patients with PTMC remains to be defined.[11]

Another area of considerable controversy in surgical management of DTC is whether or not to perform a prophylactic CND.[12,13] The relevance of CND for patients with clinically or radiographically evident nodes is well established. In addition, the ATA guidelines suggest that routine prophylactic CND may be performed for patients with T3 or T4 tumors, because patients with lesions 4 cm or greater have an increased risk of nodal metastases[4]; however, for patients with tumors less than 4 cm, the evidence for prophylactic CND is less clear. Many patients with PTC with clinically node-negative disease undergoing prophylactic CND have occult positive nodes,[14–17] and prophylactic CND reduces postoperative thyroglobulin levels,[18–21] but in a recently published meta-analysis, CND was not associated with a significant decrease in local recurrence.[22] Prophylactic CND does seem to increase postoperative morbidity,[14,19] but the information obtained from prophylactic CND may provide important staging information, because lymph node status was an independent predictor of survival in a recent study of the SEER database.[23] Clearly, this is an area in need of further study to effectively define which patients most benefit from CND.

HISTORICAL PERSPECTIVE

Thyroid surgery has seen many advances over the years. Thyroid disease has been recognized throughout much of human history, beginning with early writings from China regarding the use of seaweed to treat goiter in 2700 BC.[24] Early thyroid operations, before the advent of modern techniques and asepsis, were performed largely only because of morbidity associated with goiters causing airway obstruction. Dr Samuel Gross wrote in 1866, "every step the surgeon takes will be environed with difficulty; every stroke of his knife will be followed by a torrent of blood, and lucky will it be for him if his victim lives long enough to enable him to finish his horrid butchery."[24] Because of the early difficulty with thyroidectomy, it is not surprising that some of the most recognized surgeons in history made significant advances in thyroid surgery, including Theodor Billroth, Theodor Kocher, William Steward Halsted, and Charles Mayo.[25] Dr Kocher was awarded the 1909 Nobel Prize for Medicine for his pioneering work in thyroid physiology and surgery. The legacy of innovation and progress in thyroid surgery has continued through the modern era. Currently, this innovation is most notable in the form of minimally invasive techniques for the treatment of thyroid disease and thyroid cancer. In this article, the application of these techniques is discussed, including endoscopic and robotic surgery for thyroid disease.

Early advances in minimally invasive, or less-invasive, techniques of thyroid surgery involved using smaller open incisions, evolving from 8-cm to 10-cm incisions to the use of 3-cm to 5-cm incisions.[26] The introduction and widespread adoption of endoscopic technology then led to the use of this technology in thyroid surgery. Although the open approach is expeditious, and the incision is generally well hidden in a cervical neck crease, possible advantages of endoscopic approaches include improved cosmesis and, given the use of endoscopes with magnification, potentially improved visualization. Currently, several different methods of endoscopic approach to the thyroid gland are practiced, and we review the different techniques and the current literature about these various approaches (**Table 1**).

ENDOSCOPIC THYROIDECTOMY

The first endoscopic thyroid surgery was reported by Huscher and colleagues,[27] when they described the use of an anterior cervical approach to perform a right thyroid lobectomy. This lobectomy was accomplished using 3-mm to 5-mm ports. One port was at the jugular notch, one was at the angle of the mandible, and one was midway between the other 2. These investigators used a 30° endoscope and CO_2 insufflation to develop a dissection plane in the subplatysmal space. Since this initial description, various other techniques for endoscopic removal of the thyroid have been described. The most commonly used procedure in North America is the minimally invasive video-assisted thyroidectomy (MIVAT). This procedure was initially described for the treatment of small thyroid nodules in 1999 by Miccoli and colleagues.[28] Several alternative approaches to endoscopic thyroidectomy have been described as well. The transaxillary approach was initially described in 2001 by Ikeda and colleagues[29] for unilateral thyroid lesions and has been adopted by some groups, both unilaterally and bilaterally, for endoscopic as well as robotic thyroidectomy. In addition, various other extracervical approaches have been described, some as combinations of other techniques. These approaches include an anterior chest approach,[30] a breast approach,[31,32] and the axillobilateral breast approach (ABBA).[33,34] Feasibility and limited clinical studies have also been described using a retroauricular approach,[35] a dorsal approach,[36] and a transoral, incisionless approach for both endoscopic[37,38] and robotic thyroidectomy.[39] Here we discuss some of the technical aspects of the most commonly used cervical techniques (the MIVAT approach), as well as some aspects of the more widely used extracervical techniques including the transaxillary approach.

The MIVAT approach, as originally described for thyroid lobectomy, is accomplished by first making a 15-mm incision 2 cm superior to the sternal notch, followed by careful dissection in the subplatysmal plane. The linea alba is then incised for approximately 3 to 4 cm. A 12-mm trocar is then introduced between the strap muscles and the thyroid lobe, and CO_2 insufflation is applied under direct visualization with a 30° 5-mm endoscope to 12 mm Hg for approximately 3 minutes to further develop the dissection plane between the thyroid and the strap muscles, opening the thyrotracheal groove. After this time, insufflation is allowed to fully egress. Needle-scopic 2-mm forceps and aspirator are then introduced under direct visualization through a small supraclavicular incision and 2-mm scissors or a spatula are introduced through the main incision. The dissection is then carried out laterally to medially,

Table 1
Summary of access points and camera position for different methods of completing endoscopic and robotic thyroidectomy

Technique	Year	Port Sites	Camera Position	References
Minimally invasive video-assisted thyroidectomy	1999	1. 2 cm above sternal notch: 12 mm 2. 1 cm above clavicle: 2 mm instruments	Suprasternal	28
Endoscopic breast approach	2000	1. Ipsilateral parasternal: 12 mm 2. Bilateral supra-areolar: 1 x 5 mm in each site	Ipsilateral parasternal	31
Endoscopic transaxillary approach	2001	1. Ipsilateral (or bilateral) axilla: 6-cm incision with 3-4 ports	Axilla	29
Endoscopic anterior chest approach	2002	1. Inferior ipsilateral clavicle: 12 mm 2. Inferior ipsilateral clavicle: 5 mm 3. Inferior sternal notch: 5 mm	Inferior ipsilateral clavicle	30
Endoscopic axillobilateral breast approach	2003	1. Bilateral axilla: 1 x l0 mm in each axilla 2. Bilateral supra-areolar: 1 x 5 mm in each site	Axilla	33
Robotic anterior chest axillary approach	2009	1. Axilla: 6-cm incision with 3 ports 2. Medial anterior chest: 5 mm	Axilla	60
Robotic bilateral axillary bilateral areolar approach	2009	1. Bilateral axillary: 1 x 8-12 mm in each axilla 2. Bilateral supra-areolar: 1 x 8-12 mm in each site	Right supra-areolar	63
Robotic unilateral transaxillary approach	2010	1. Axilla: 6-cm incision, 4 ports	Axilla	59
Robotic retroauricular face-lift incision approach	2011	1. Postauricular crease: 3 arms	Postauricular crease	64

carefully identifying the parathyroid glands and recurrent laryngeal nerve (RLN). Bipolar cautery is used for hemostasis on smaller vessels away from the RLN and clips are used on larger vessels and those near the RLN. Once the thyroid is mobilized from these important structures, the dissection is carried out in standard fashion, removing the gland from the trachea. To complete a lobectomy, the isthmus is then dissected and divided from the contralateral lobe by running absorbable sutures. The specimen is then removed from the main incision, hemostasis is confirmed, and the linea alba and platysma are closed with absorbable sutures. Generally, no drains are left in place.[40] The generally accepted indications for MIVAT are as follows: benign thyroid nodules, the largest diameter of which is less than 35 mm, cytologically malignant nodules less than 20 mm, and an ultrasonographically estimated thyroid volume less than 25 cm^3.[41] It is also believed that the presence of either severe thyroiditis, or preoperative suspicion of metastasis to either the lateral or central neck lymph nodes, are contraindications to performing MIVAT; however, it has been recently suggested that these contraindications may be unfounded. In a series of nearly 2000 patients (511 thyroid lobectomy, 1435 total thyroidectomy) recently published by Minuto and colleagues,[41] it was found that up to 30% of patients with PTC had thyroiditis on final pathologic examination and only 1 case was converted to open because of thyroiditis. In addition, these investigators found that the mean number of nodes removed in patients with suspected central neck metastases was similar to the number removed in open operations in their hands.[41,42]

The transaxillary endoscopic approach to thyroidectomy was originally developed to provide a safe operative approach for patients concerned with the cosmesis of a neck incision.[29] The patient is positioned with arm(s) out depending on the affected side or bilaterality of the operation. Generally, a 1.5-cm to 3-cm incision is made in the axilla and the platysma is exposed through the upper portion of the pectoralis major muscle or via tunneling subcutaneously. Conventional 12-mm and 5-mm trocars are placed in the axillary incision, the trocars are then purse-stringed in place, and a low insufflation pressure (3–6 mm Hg) is applied for a few minutes. After adequate insufflation is achieved, 1 to 2 additional ports are placed in the axilla to allow access for dissection instruments. The thyroid is then exposed by dissection of the sternocleidomastoid from the strap muscles (sternohyoid and sternothyroid). The thyroid dissection then progresses as described earlier, with careful identification of the RLN and superior and inferior parathyroid glands. Once the thyroid has been sufficiently mobilized and the key structures identified, the thyroid is then dissected off the trachea, and the isthmus is transected using the harmonic scalpel for completion of a lobectomy. The specimen is then extracted via the main axillary incision, a closed suction drain is left in the subplatysmal space, and the skin is closed in standard fashion.[29] Modifications of this approach that include breast incisions (Refs.[33,34] ABBA) typically use bilateral superior areolar incisions. In the ABBA approach, the endoscope is typically inserted via one of the areolar incisions and most of the dissection is accomplished via instruments introduced through the axillary incision(s).

COMPARING OPEN AND ENDOSCOPIC THYROIDECTOMY

As discussed earlier, the main driving force for minimally invasive thyroidectomy is improved cosmesis. A recent meta-analysis looked at the available prospective trials comparing MIVAT versus conventional open thyroidectomy.[43] The primary end points of this study were postoperative pain, hypocalcemia, and RLN injury. Early postoperative pain was consistently decreased in patients treated with MIVAT,[44–48] and there were no differences in postoperative hypocalcemia or RLN injury.[43] In addition, a recent cost-effectiveness study showed a shorter hospital stay for patients after MIVAT with similar operative costs,[49] belying the premise that open thyroidectomy is more cost-effective. However, this study had postoperative average hospital stays of 1.16 days versus 1.62 days, the clinical significance of which is unclear. Further evaluation of MIVAT and conventional thyroidectomy via an adequately powered randomized controlled trial is warranted to establish noninferiority for postsurgical morbidity and oncologic outcomes as well as improved subjective patient outcomes, including cosmesis and pain. Other smaller studies have also been published corroborating the data in this meta-analysis and randomized trials[50,51]

There are also several reports comparing the transaxillary approach and the ABBA approach with conventional thyroidectomy, primarily from groups outside the United States, where this technique is more commonly used. Initially, Ikeda and colleagues,[52] who originally described the transaxillary approach, used both the transaxillary and combination axillary and anterior chest approach and published their results in a small study comparing both endoscopic methods and the standard open approach. In this study, both endoscopic methods took significantly longer than the open approach (175 minutes vs 145 minutes vs 84 minutes, respectively) and patients undergoing endoscopic thyroidectomy experienced similar short-term pain and less long-term neck hypesthesia than those undergoing conventional thyroidectomy. However, patients undergoing combined transaxillary and anterior chest endoscopic resection had worse subjective satisfaction with cosmesis 3 months postoperatively, leading this group to focus on the transaxillary approach.[52] In a subsequent study, Ikeda and colleagues[53] published their initial results in a small group of patients undergoing total thyroidectomy via the transaxillary approach (20 open and 20 endoscopic) in 2003 and showed again that operative times were significantly longer in the endoscopic group and that patients treated endoscopically had a nonsignificant increase in overall pain scores in the immediate postoperative period, resolving by 4 days after surgery. However, increased anterior chest pain was consistently expressed by patients undergoing endoscopic resection, whereas no patients in the open group complained of this pain. Despite increased pain scores at 3 months after surgery, patients were significantly more satisfied with cosmesis after transaxillary resection. Other groups have published their results using both the transaxillary and ABBA approaches, with varying results. Consistently across all studies, operative times were increased for patients undergoing endoscopic thyroidectomy, immediate postoperative pain scores were similar or reduced, and subjective cosmesis was believed to be improved by patients at 3 months after surgery in the endoscopic groups.[54-57] However, some studies have reported increased postoperative complications, including transient RLN palsy[56,57] and transient hypocalcemia.[56] In addition, local recurrence of a follicular neoplasm in a port tract has been reported after transaxillary thyroidectomy.[58] It seems that in experienced hands, the transaxillary approach is a safe procedure in patients who desire to avoid a cervical incision; however, there are not enough data to recommend widespread adoption of this technique.

ROBOTIC THYROIDECTOMY

As more groups have gained experience with endoscopic approaches to the thyroid and robotic technology has advanced, the application of robotic technology to thyroidectomy was a logical next step. The potential advantages of robotic thyroidectomy over endoscopic thyroidectomy include the ability to perform more precise dissection because of the dexterity afforded by the robot, improved visualization because of three-dimensional magnification and surgeon-controlled visualization and a hand tremor filtering system.[59,60] The first large series of robotic thyroidectomy was reported in 2009 by Kang and colleagues,[60] who used a combination of a unilateral transaxillary incision and an anterior chest incision for both benign thyroid disease as well as for PTC (**Fig. 1**).[61,62] Also in 2009, a robotic bilateral axillary, bilateral areolar approach was described.[63] In 2010, a single-incision transaxillary approach was described to alleviate some of the anterior chest symptoms experienced with the addition of the anterior chest access.[59] Recently, an alternative, nonaxillary approach has been described using a retroauricular face-lift incision, which may avoid the potential added morbidity from an axillary incision.[64] An important consideration regarding robotic thyroidectomy is that there is a considerable learning curve. Kang and colleagues[62] reported in their original series a significant decrease in console operating time after 40 to 50 cases, although significant fluctuations remained even after the first 50 cases. One published study looked prospectively at the difference between an experienced surgeon (>50 cases) and 3 surgeons with experience in endoscopic but not robotic thyroidectomy as well as the learning curve for these surgeons.[65] This group corroborated the findings that after 50 cases, operative times significantly improved. The first 50 total thyroidectomies took inexperienced surgeons an average of 181.5 minutes to complete (from first incision to closure); however, subsequent cases after 50 took these surgeons an average of 141.5 minutes, which was similar to the experienced surgeon (132.8 minutes). In addition, this group also looked at complications in relation to the learning curve. In 267 cases performed by the experienced surgeon there were no major complications, including permanent RLN injury, whereas there were 9 major complications (5 permanent RLN, 2 permanent hypocalcemia, 1 hematoma with reoperation, 1 tracheal injury) in 377 patients undergoing operation by inexperienced surgeons. Most of these complications occurred in the

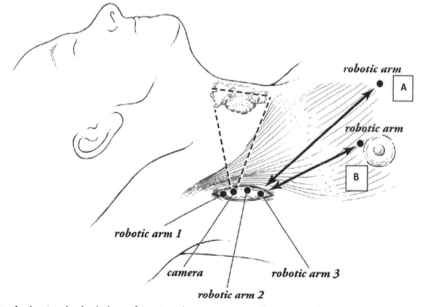

Fig. 1. Anatomic depiction of port and camera access for transaxillary robotic thyroidectomy. Different groups have described using anterior chest (A) or breast (B) access points for a third robotic arm.

first 50 cases. Minor complications were similar in both groups. One series of 100 operations, most of which were thyroid lobectomy, by 1 surgeon in North America has been described, and in this series there is also a significant decrease in average operative time after 45 cases.[66] There was only 1 major complication in this study, which occurred in the first 45 cases. This group also looked at the effect of body mass index (BMI, calculated as weight in kilograms divided by the square of height in meters) on operative time and found a significantly increased operative time in patients with BMI greater than 30 (137.1 vs 99.7 minutes), lending credence to the assertion that this modality may be less applicable to overweight and obese patients.

COMPARING OPEN AND ROBOTIC THYROIDECTOMY

Two recent studies have been published comparing outcomes between the open technique and the transaxillary robotic technique. Foley and colleagues[67] published a small prospective case series, in which they found no difference in surgical outcomes between patients undergoing robotic or open thyroidectomy, albeit with a significantly longer operative time (232 vs 109 minutes, respectively) and incision length (6 vs 3.6 cm, respectively) in the robotic group. A larger retrospective study from Yonsei University in Korea, including more than 400 patients, has also recently been published, which showed similar surgical outcomes in terms of oncologic resection and complications between open and robotic thyroidectomy.[59] However, in this study, the extent of surgical resection was different in the 2 groups, in that patients undergoing robotic thyroidectomy were more likely to have undergone subtotal thyroidectomy than patients undergoing open surgery. In addition, the robotic group were more likely to have bilateral lesions and were more likely to be female; therefore it is difficult to make concrete conclusions from this study.

COMPARING ENDOSCOPIC AND ROBOTIC THYROIDECTOMY

An important consideration for the application of robotic technology is whether it truly adds benefits when compared with traditional endoscopic techniques. A few groups have looked at outcomes comparing the 2 techniques in an attempt to shed some light on this important clinical question. In a retrospective review of their experience with conventional endoscopic and robotic thyroidectomy using the transaxillary method with the addition of an anterior chest port, Lee and colleagues[65] found that endoscopic thyroidectomy took significantly longer and had a longer learning curve; however, there was no difference in complications. However, this study primarily involved patients with tumors less than 10 mm, and there were important differences between the 2 groups. Patients undergoing robotic thyroidectomy in this study were significantly more likely to have a total instead of a subtotal thyroidectomy and a diagnosis of cancer. In another small study involving approximately 200 patients, Yoo and colleagues[68] found similar disparities among patients undergoing robotic and endoscopic thyroidectomy, including a larger percentage of patients undergoing total thyroidectomy in the robotic group. However, when they compared operative times, these investigators found that for each procedure (either thyroid lobectomy or total thyroidectomy), the endoscopic procedure was significantly shorter. They also found that postoperative length of stay and complications were similar between the 2 groups. They also commented on the cost of surgery and noted that the cost of robotic thyroidectomy was 8 times as costly as endoscopic thyroidectomy ($6655 vs $829, respectively). In a larger study including more than 1000 patients, the group from Yonsei University in Korea published their experience with the transaxillary with anterior chest port technique in the setting of PTMC.[69] In this study, it was again found that significantly more patients underwent total thyroidectomy in the robotic group and patients had significantly more advanced tumors; however, operative times were similar, as well as rates of complication, with the exception of transient hypocalcemia, which was more common among patients undergoing robotic thyroidectomy. These studies again seem to confirm that both endoscopic and robotic thyroidectomy are procedures that can be performed safely, with good outcomes in appropriately selected patients. However, it is difficult to draw definitive conclusions from these data regarding whether either technique is superior to the other, and future study may be warranted.

SUMMARY AND FUTURE DIRECTIONS

As technology advances, application of new technologies continues to be an important issue in all fields of surgery, and thyroid surgery is no exception. Sufficient data suggest that endoscopic and robotic surgery can be applied safely in at least a subset of patients with thyroid disease. Given the wide variety of techniques being evaluated, and the proven efficacy, cost-effectiveness, and high patient satisfaction associated with standard surgical techniques, additional study is warranted to determine the applicability of endoscopic and robotic thyroidectomy in the treatment of patients with thyroid disease.

REFERENCES

1. Siegel R, Naishadham D, Jemal A. Cancer statistics. CA Cancer J Clin 2012; 62(1):10–29.
2. Simard EP, Ward EM, Siegel R, et al. Cancers with increasing incidence trends in the United States: 1999 through 2008. CA Cancer J Clin 2012;62(2):118–28.
3. Davies L, Welch HG. Increasing incidence of thyroid cancer in the United States, 1973-2002. JAMA 2006;295(18):2164–7.
4. Cooper DS, Doherty GM, Haugen BR, et al. Revised American Thyroid Association management guidelines for patients with thyroid nodules and differentiated thyroid cancer. Thyroid 2009;19(11):1167–214.
5. Bilimoria KY, Bentrem DJ, Ko CY, et al. Extent of surgery affects survival for papillary thyroid cancer. Ann Surg 2007;246(3):375–81 [discussion: 381–74].
6. Barney BM, Hitchcock YJ, Sharma P, et al. Overall and cause-specific survival for patients undergoing lobectomy, near-total, or total thyroidectomy for differentiated thyroid cancer. Head Neck 2011;33(5):645–9.
7. Mazeh H, Samet Y, Hochstein D, et al. Multifocality in well-differentiated thyroid carcinomas calls for total thyroidectomy. Am J Surg 2011;201(6):770–5.
8. Pitt SC, Sippel RS, Chen H. Contralateral papillary thyroid cancer: does size matter? Am J Surg 2009;197(3):342–7.
9. Hay ID, Hutchinson ME, Gonzalez-Losada T, et al. Papillary thyroid microcarcinoma: a study of 900 cases observed in a 60-year period. Surgery 2008;144(6):980–7 [discussion: 987–8].
10. Chow SM, Law SC, Chan JK, et al. Papillary microcarcinoma of the thyroid–prognostic significance of lymph node metastasis and multifocality. Cancer 2003; 98(1):31–40.
11. Yu XM, Wan Y, Sippel RS, et al. Should all papillary thyroid microcarcinomas be aggressively treated? An analysis of 18,445 cases. Ann Surg 2011;254(4):653–60.
12. Mazzaferri EL, Doherty GM, Steward DL. The pros and cons of prophylactic central compartment lymph node dissection for papillary thyroid carcinoma. Thyroid 2009;19(7):683–9.

13. Roh JL, Kim JM, Park CI. Central lymph node metastasis of unilateral papillary thyroid carcinoma: patterns and factors predictive of nodal metastasis, morbidity, and recurrence. Ann Surg Oncol 2011;18(8):2245–50.
14. Palestini N, Borasi A, Cestino L, et al. Is central neck dissection a safe procedure in the treatment of papillary thyroid cancer? Our experience. Langenbecks Arch Surg 2008;393(5):693–8.
15. Hyun SM, Song HY, Kim SY, et al. Impact of combined prophylactic unilateral central neck dissection and hemithyroidectomy in patients with papillary thyroid microcarcinoma. Ann Surg Oncol 2012;19(2):591–6.
16. Pereira JA, Jimeno J, Miquel J, et al. Nodal yield, morbidity, and recurrence after central neck dissection for papillary thyroid carcinoma. Surgery 2005;138(6): 1095–100 [discussion: 1100–091].
17. Bozec A, Dassonville O, Chamorey E, et al. Clinical impact of cervical lymph node involvement and central neck dissection in patients with papillary thyroid carcinoma: a retrospective analysis of 368 cases. Eur Arch Otorhinolaryngol 2011;268(8):1205–12.
18. Sywak M, Cornford L, Roach P, et al. Routine ipsilateral level VI lymphadenectomy reduces postoperative thyroglobulin levels in papillary thyroid cancer. Surgery 2006;140(6):1000–5 [discussion: 1005–7].
19. So YK, Seo MY, Son YI. Prophylactic central lymph node dissection for clinically node-negative papillary thyroid microcarcinoma: influence on serum thyroglobulin level, recurrence rate, and postoperative complications. Surgery 2012; 151(2):192–8.
20. Lang BH, Wong KP, Wan KY, et al. Impact of routine unilateral central neck dissection on preablative and postablative stimulated thyroglobulin levels after total thyroidectomy in papillary thyroid carcinoma. Ann Surg Oncol 2012;19(1): 60–7.
21. Popadich A, Levin O, Lee JC, et al. A multicenter cohort study of total thyroidectomy and routine central lymph node dissection for cN0 papillary thyroid cancer. Surgery 2011;150(6):1048–57.
22. Zetoune T, Keutgen X, Buitrago D, et al. Prophylactic central neck dissection and local recurrence in papillary thyroid cancer: a meta-analysis. Ann Surg Oncol 2010;17(12):3287–93.
23. Podnos YD, Smith D, Wagman LD, et al. The implication of lymph node metastasis on survival in patients with well-differentiated thyroid cancer. Am Surg 2005;71(9):731–4.
24. Rogers-Stevane J, Kauffman GL Jr. A historical perspective on surgery of the thyroid and parathyroid glands. Otolaryngol Clin North Am 2008;41(6):1059–67, vii.
25. Sakorafas GH. Historical evolution of thyroid surgery: from the ancient times to the dawn of the 21st century. World J Surg 2010;34(8):1793–804.
26. Brunaud L, Zarnegar R, Wada N, et al. Incision length for standard thyroidectomy and parathyroidectomy: when is it minimally invasive? Arch Surg 2003;138(10): 1140–3.
27. Huscher CS, Chiodini S, Napolitano C, et al. Endoscopic right thyroid lobectomy. Surg Endosc 1997;11(8):877.
28. Miccoli P, Berti P, Conte M, et al. Minimally invasive surgery for thyroid small nodules: preliminary report. J Endocrinol Invest 1999;22(11):849–51.
29. Ikeda Y, Takami H, Niimi M, et al. Endoscopic thyroidectomy by the axillary approach. Surg Endosc 2001;15(11):1362–4.
30. Ikeda Y, Takami H, Tajima G, et al. Total endoscopic thyroidectomy: axillary or anterior chest approach. Biomed Pharmacother 2002;56(Suppl 1):72s–8s.

31. Ohgami M, Ishii S, Arisawa Y, et al. Scarless endoscopic thyroidectomy: breast approach for better cosmesis. Surg Laparosc Endosc Percutan Tech 2000; 10(1):1–4.
32. Hur SM, Kim SH, Lee SK, et al. New endoscopic thyroidectomy with the bilateral areolar approach: a comparison with the bilateral axillo-breast approach. Surg Laparosc Endosc Percutan Tech 2011;21(5):e219–24.
33. Barlehner E, Benhidjeb T. Cervical scarless endoscopic thyroidectomy: axillo-bilateral-breast approach (ABBA). Surg Endosc 2008;22(1):154–7.
34. Shimazu K, Shiba E, Tamaki Y, et al. Endoscopic thyroid surgery through the axillo-bilateral-breast approach. Surg Laparosc Endosc Percutan Tech 2003; 13(3):196–201.
35. Walvekar RR, Wallace E, Bergeron B, et al. Retro-auricular video-assisted "gas-less" thyroidectomy: feasibility study in human cadavers. Surg Endosc 2010; 24(11):2895–9.
36. Schardey HM, Schopf S, Kammal M, et al. Invisible scar endoscopic thyroidectomy by the dorsal approach: experimental development of a new technique with human cadavers and preliminary clinical results. Surg Endosc 2008;22(4): 813–20.
37. Witzel K, von Rahden BH, Kaminski C, et al. Transoral access for endoscopic thyroid resection. Surg Endosc 2008;22(8):1871–5.
38. Benhidjeb T, Wilhelm T, Harlaar J, et al. Natural orifice surgery on thyroid gland: totally transoral video-assisted thyroidectomy (TOVAT): report of first experimental results of a new surgical method. Surg Endosc 2009;23(5):1119–20.
39. Richmon JD, Pattani KM, Benhidjeb T, et al. Transoral robotic-assisted thyroidectomy: a preclinical feasibility study in 2 cadavers. Head Neck 2011;33(3):330–3.
40. Miccoli P, Berti P, Bendinelli C, et al. Minimally invasive video-assisted surgery of the thyroid: a preliminary report. Langenbecks Arch Surg 2000;385(4):261–4.
41. Minuto MN, Berti P, Miccoli M, et al. Minimally invasive video-assisted thyroidectomy: an analysis of results and a revision of indications. Surg Endosc 2012; 26(3):818–22.
42. Miccoli P, Minuto MN, Ugolini C, et al. Clinically unpredictable prognostic factors in the outcome of medullary thyroid cancer. Endocr Relat Cancer 2007;14(4): 1099–105.
43. Radford PD, Ferguson MS, Magill JC, et al. Meta-analysis of minimally invasive video-assisted thyroidectomy. Laryngoscope 2011;121(8):1675–81.
44. Miccoli P, Berti P, Raffaelli M, et al. Comparison between minimally invasive video-assisted thyroidectomy and conventional thyroidectomy: a prospective randomized study. Surgery 2001;130(6):1039–43.
45. Bellantone R, Lombardi CP, Bossola M, et al. Video-assisted vs conventional thyroid lobectomy: a randomized trial. Arch Surg 2002;137(3):301–4 [discussion 305].
46. Chao TC, Lin JD, Chen MF. Video-assisted open thyroid lobectomy through a small incision. Surg Laparosc Endosc Percutan Tech 2004;14(1):15–9.
47. Lombardi CP, Raffaelli M, Princi P, et al. Safety of video-assisted thyroidectomy versus conventional surgery. Head Neck 2005;27(1):58–64.
48. El-Labban GM. Minimally invasive video-assisted thyroidectomy versus conventional thyroidectomy: a single-blinded, randomized controlled clinical trial. J Minim Access Surg 2009;5(4):97–102.
49. Byrd JK, Nguyen SA, Ketcham A, et al. Minimally invasive video-assisted thyroidectomy versus conventional thyroidectomy: a cost-effective analysis. Otolaryngol Head Neck Surg 2010;143(6):789–94.

50. Dobrinja C, Trevisan G, Makovac P, et al. Minimally invasive video-assisted thyroidectomy compared with conventional thyroidectomy in a general surgery department. Surg Endosc 2009;23(10):2263–7.

51. Del Rio P, Berti M, Sommaruga L, et al. Pain after minimally invasive videoassisted and after minimally invasive open thyroidectomy–results of a prospective outcome study. Langenbecks Arch Surg 2008;393(3):271–3.

52. Ikeda Y, Takami H, Niimi M, et al. Endoscopic thyroidectomy and parathyroidectomy by the axillary approach. A preliminary report. Surg Endosc 2002;16(1): 92–5.

53. Ikeda Y, Takami H, Sasaki Y, et al. Clinical benefits in endoscopic thyroidectomy by the axillary approach. J Am Coll Surg 2003;196(2):189–95.

54. Tae K, Ji YB, Cho SH, et al. Initial experience with a gasless unilateral axillo-breast or axillary approach endoscopic thyroidectomy for papillary thyroid microcarcinoma: comparison with conventional open thyroidectomy. Surg Laparosc Endosc Percutan Tech 2011;21(3):162–9.

55. Jiang ZG, Zhang W, Jiang DZ, et al. Clinical benefits of scarless endoscopic thyroidectomy: an expert's experience. World J Surg 2011;35(3):553–7.

56. Jeong JJ, Kang SW, Yun JS, et al. Comparative study of endoscopic thyroidectomy versus conventional open thyroidectomy in papillary thyroid microcarcinoma (PTMC) patients. J Surg Oncol 2009;100(6):477–80.

57. Chung YS, Choe JH, Kang KH, et al. Endoscopic thyroidectomy for thyroid malignancies: comparison with conventional open thyroidectomy. World J Surg 2007; 31(12):2302–6 [discussion: 2307–8].

58. Beninato T, Kleiman DA, Scognamiglio T, et al. Tract recurrence of a follicular thyroid neoplasm following transaxillary endoscopic thyroidectomy. Thyroid 2012;22(2):214–7.

59. Ryu HR, Kang SW, Lee SH, et al. Feasibility and safety of a new robotic thyroidectomy through a gasless, transaxillary single-incision approach. J Am Coll Surg 2010;211(3):e13–9.

60. Kang SW, Jeong JJ, Yun JS, et al. Robot-assisted endoscopic surgery for thyroid cancer: experience with the first 100 patients. Surg Endosc 2009;23(11): 2399–406.

61. Kang SW, Jeong JJ, Nam KH, et al. Robot-assisted endoscopic thyroidectomy for thyroid malignancies using a gasless transaxillary approach. J Am Coll Surg 2009;209(2):e1–7.

62. Kang SW, Lee SC, Lee SH, et al. Robotic thyroid surgery using a gasless, transaxillary approach and the da Vinci S system: the operative outcomes of 338 consecutive patients. Surgery 2009;146(6):1048–55.

63. Lee KE, Rao J, Youn YK. Endoscopic thyroidectomy with the da Vinci robot system using the bilateral axillary breast approach (BABA) technique: our initial experience. Surg Laparosc Endosc Percutan Tech 2009;19(3):e71–5.

64. Terris DJ, Singer MC, Seybt MW. Robotic facelift thyroidectomy: patient selection and technical considerations. Surg Laparosc Endosc Percutan Tech 2011;21(4): 237–42.

65. Lee J, Lee JH, Nah KY, et al. Comparison of endoscopic and robotic thyroidectomy. Ann Surg Oncol 2011;18(5):1439–46.

66. Kandil EH, Noureldine SI, Yao L, et al. Robotic transaxillary thyroidectomy: an examination of the first one hundred cases. J Am Coll Surg 2012;214(4):558–64.

67. Foley CS, Agcaoglu O, Siperstein AE, et al. Robotic transaxillary endocrine surgery: a comparison with conventional open technique. Surg Endosc 2012; 26(8):2259–66.

68. Yoo H, Chae BJ, Park HS, et al. Comparison of surgical outcomes between endoscopic and robotic thyroidectomy. J Surg Oncol 2012;105(7):705–8.
69. Lee S, Ryu HR, Park JH, et al. Excellence in robotic thyroid surgery: a comparative study of robot-assisted versus conventional endoscopic thyroidectomy in papillary thyroid microcarcinoma patients. Ann Surg 2011;253(6):1060–6.

Minimally Invasive Surgery for Esophageal Cancer

Christian G. Peyre, MD, Jeffrey H. Peters, MD*

KEYWORDS

- Minimally invasive esophagectomy • Esophageal cancer
- Minimally invasive surgery • Esophagectomy

KEY POINTS

- Esophagectomy remains the best curative treatment of resectable esophageal cancer.
- Minimally invasive surgery has revolutionized the surgical management of benign foregut disease, and pulmonary and other gastrointestinal malignancies, and is gaining popularity in the management of esophageal cancer.
- The important principles and techniques of minimally invasive esophagectomy are described in this article.
- Minimally invasive esophagectomy has short-term results equivalent to those of open resection, with comparable morbidity and mortality, and some reports demonstrate a decreased rate of cardiopulmonary complications.
- Long-term oncologic results for minimally invasive esophagectomy are unclear. The number of resected lymph nodes is comparable with that reported for open surgery, but locoregional recurrence rate and long-term survival needs to be studied.

INTRODUCTION

Esophagectomy remains the best curative option for the treatment of resectable esophageal cancer, but is a complex operation with significant morbidity and mortality. Over the past decade, minimally invasive esophagectomy (MIE) has been gaining favor as an attractive alternative to open resection with the potential to reduce surgical trauma, decrease morbidity, and shorten the length of hospital stay.[1] While minimally invasive surgery has revolutionized pulmonary surgery, treatment of benign foregut disease, and management of other gastrointestinal malignancies, adoption of MIE has been slow. The aim of this article is to review the technique and results of MIE for esophageal cancer.

Department of Surgery, University of Rochester School of Medicine & Dentistry, 601 Elmwood Avenue, BOX SURG, Rochester, NY 14642, USA
* Corresponding author.
E-mail address: Jeffrey_Peters@urmc.rochester.edu

Surg Oncol Clin N Am 22 (2013) 15–25
http://dx.doi.org/10.1016/j.soc.2012.08.010
1055-3207/13/$ – see front matter © 2013 Elsevier Inc. All rights reserved.

HISTORY OF MINIMALLY INVASIVE ESOPHAGECTOMY

Beginning with the first successful esophageal resection by Torek in 1913, esophagectomy has undergone considerable refinement and evolution over the past century. Despite decades of experience, controversy remains as to the optimal open surgical technique for resection of the esophagus and reconstruction of the alimentary tract. Debated issues include the oncologic benefits of a transthoracic versus transhiatal resection and the relative risk of constructing the anastomosis in the neck or chest.

The late 1980s ushered in the modern era of minimally invasive surgery. Techniques and instruments were developed for laparoscopic and video-assisted thoracoscopic surgery (VATS). Over the ensuing 2 decades, minimally invasive surgery for gastroesophageal reflux, paraesophageal hernias, achalasia, obesity, colon cancer, and lung cancer have become standardized and have supplanted open surgery as the standard operation.

As experience in minimally invasive surgery grew, initial attempts at esophageal resection were undertaken. In 1993, Collard and colleagues[2] published their initial experience with thoracoscopic mobilization of the esophagus. In 1995, DePaula and colleagues[3] published an early clinical series of their experience with laparoscopic transhiatal esophagectomy. By the late 1990s initial reports of combined thoracoscopic and laparoscopic esophagectomy and reconstruction were being published, documenting the feasibility of the operation.[4,5] Despite the great enthusiasm to adopt minimally invasive surgery for other intrathoracic or intra-abdominal diseases, MIE has been slow to be adopted and only accounts for about 15% of all esophagectomies performed.[6]

RATIONALE FOR MINIMALLY INVASIVE ESOPHAGECTOMY

The advent and refinement of minimally invasive surgery has been a transformative event in surgical science. Worldwide acceptance by clinicians and patients has been driven by improved outcomes and patient satisfaction over open surgery. Classic examples include the tremendous increase in popularity of laparoscopic obesity surgery and laparoscopic cholecystectomy for benign gallbladder disease.

Treatment of benign foregut disease has been revolutionized by minimally invasive surgery. Before laparoscopy, surgical treatment of gastroesophageal reflux disease was reserved for those patients with severe, uncontrollable symptoms and complications from long-standing disease (ie, strictures) due to the morbidity associated with open repair.[7] Beginning in 1991, the technique of laparoscopic Nissen fundoplication was developed, and the operation is now a reasonable alternative to medical therapy even in patients with moderate disease.[8,9] In addition, laparoscopy has nearly eliminated the need for transthoracic antireflux operations. Laparoscopic antireflux surgery is an extremely safe operation with low mortality and morbidity. A recent analysis of a nationwide database in the United States found the mortality following laparoscopic Nissen fundoplication to be extremely low.[10] Complication rates, length of hospital stay, and patient satisfaction are significantly improved in comparison with open surgery.[11] Similarly, laparoscopic paraesophageal hernia repair and laparoscopic Heller myotomy have become the standard operations for the management of large paraesophageal hernias and achalasia.

With the popularity of minimally invasive surgery for benign disease well established, adoption of a minimally invasive approach for oncologic surgery was initially approached with trepidation out of concern for compromised oncologic outcomes and port-site recurrences. Despite initial concerns, multiple trials for both intrathoracic and intra-abdominal malignancies have reported the early benefits of minimally invasive surgery but have also demonstrated oncologic equivalence. Trials in colon cancer and lung cancer have shown equivalent lymph node harvest, and ability to achieve complete R0 resection and long-term survival.[12,13] In many centers, laparoscopic colectomy and VATS lobectomy are standard of care for the management of most colon and pulmonary malignancies.

Mortality following open esophagectomy ranges from 2% to 8% in experienced centers and can be as high as 15% to 20% in low-volume centers.[14] Complications following open esophageal resection are common. As a consequence, some centers promote definitive chemoradiotherapy to avoid the risk of resection.[15] Traditionally, pulmonary complications are the major source of morbidity following esophagectomy and are attributed to the thoracotomy and its negative impact on pain, atelectasis, and postoperative pulmonary toilet.[16] Similarly, laparotomy can have a significant negative impact on respiratory function, as pulmonary complications are common even after transhiatal resections.

With the established popularity of minimally invasive surgery, the demonstrated equivalence of minimally invasive surgery for oncologic resection, and the potential to improve the morbidity following open esophagectomy, the minimally invasive approach to esophageal resection and reconstruction may be a prudent alternative to open resection.

SURGICAL TECHNIQUE

As with open esophagectomy, there are multiple approaches to performing an MIE. Transhiatal, Ivor-Lewis, and Transthoracic (3-hole) esophagectomy are all feasible with minimally invasive techniques. The basic principles of the thoracic and abdominal dissections are similar for each surgical approach, with variations to remove of the specimen, pass the gastric conduit, and create the anastomosis.

The Thoracic Phase

The patient is intubated with a double-lumen endotracheal tube and positioned in the left lateral decubitus position for dissection in the right thoracic cavity. The patient can be rotated more prone to facilitate anterior retraction of the lung and exposure of the esophagus in the posterior mediastinum. A 4-port technique is commonly used to access the right thoracic cavity (**Fig. 1**). A camera port is positioned in the anterior

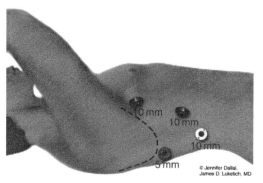

Fig. 1. Thoracoscopic port sites. (*Courtesy of* James Luketich, MD, Pittsburgh, PA. Copyright © Jennifer Dallal, MD and James Luketich, MD.)

axillary line at the seventh or eighth intercostal space. A second port is positioned in the posterior axillary line at the eighth or ninth intercostal space. These first 2 ports are placed low on the chest wall to allow dissection of the esophagus starting at the diaphragm and working cephalad. A challenging area to dissect is the costophrenic recess, which is made more difficult if ports are placed too cephalad. An axillary port is placed in the fourth intercostal space just anterior the latissimus dorsi muscle to be used by the assistant for lung retraction, suction, or countertraction of the esophagus or periesophageal tissues as needed. The fourth port is positioned just posterior to the scapular tip. The surgeon typically stands to the patient's right using primarily the posteriorly placed ports for dissection.

Once access is obtained and the lung collapsed, a fan retractor or atraumatic lung clamp can be used to retract the lung anteriorly to expose the posterior mediastinum. Additional visualization of the lower thoracic esophagus is achieved by retraction of the diaphragm using a heavy suture placed into the central tendon of the diaphragm and brought out through the camera port or a separate stab incision low on the anterolateral chest wall. Dissection of the esophagus proceeds in a caudal to cephalad direction with the aid of ultrasonic dissection. The inferior pulmonary ligament is taken down and the pleura opened in the plane anterior to the esophagus and adjacent to the pericardium. As the dissection is carried cephalad, periesophageal and subcarinal lymph nodes are dissected off the adjacent pericardium and airway en bloc with the esophagus. A plane posterior to esophagus is created just anterior to the cranially directed azygous vein. Dissection is carried down toward the aorta, which serves as the posteromedial limit of dissection. The azygous vein traversing over the esophagus toward the superior vena cava is stapled with an endoscopic linear stapler to facilitate dissection of the esophagus into the thoracic inlet.

Circumferential dissection is achieved in the mid esophagus, and a Penrose drain can be passed around the esophagus for improved retraction (**Fig. 2**). Circumferential dissection is frequently easiest just above the level of the inferior pulmonary vein where the esophagus and periesophageal tissue is dissected off the posterior pericardium. The esophagus is fully mobilized from the diaphragm to the thoracic inlet with dissection of paratracheal, subcarinal, paraesophageal, and crural lymph nodes under direct thoracoscopic guidance. Care should be taken to avoid injury to the posterior membranous wall of the trachea, which can be well visualized by the thoracoscopic camera.

Once the esophagus is fully mobilized, the Penrose drain can be loosely tied around the esophagus and positioned into the thoracic inlet, to be retrieved during the cervical phase of the operation. A second Penrose drain can be tied around the esophagus and tucked down near the diaphragm to assist in the hiatal dissection during the abdominal phase of the surgery. A single chest tube is placed and the wounds closed in the standard fashion.

The Abdominal Phase

The setup for the abdominal phase of the operation is similar to a laparoscopic Nissen fundoplication. The patient is positioned in either dorsal lithotomy or supine position with a foot rest to allow for steep reverse Trendelenburg. Typically, 5 ports are placed for a camera, liver retractor, the surgeon's dissecting ports, and a port for the assistant. With the liver retracted anteriorly, the gastrohepatic ligament is opened up to the level of the crus. If a thoracic mobilization has already been performed, dissection of the phrenoesophageal ligament and crura is delayed until the end of the abdominal phase of the operation to avoid escape of insufflated gas through the thoracic cavity. Along the greater curve of the stomach, the gastrocolic omentum and short gastric arteries

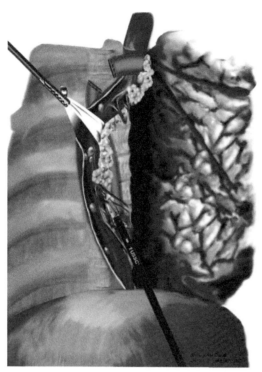

Fig. 2. Esophageal dissection facilitated by Penrose drain retraction around the esophagus. (*Courtesy of* James Luketich, MD, Pittsburgh, PA. Copyright © Jennifer Dallal, MD and James Luketich, MD.)

are divided. It is crucial to visualize the gastroepiploic arcade. Inability to adequately identify this vessel may necessitate conversion to open laparotomy to avoid injury to the critical blood supply of the gastric conduit. With the short gastrics and gastrocolic ligament mobilized, the lesser sac can be entered. Any residual adhesions to the posterior wall of the stomach and retroperitoneum are divided, and the left gastric artery is identified. After sweeping the lymphatic tissue toward the stomach, the left gastric artery is divided at its origin with a linear endoscopic stapler. The phrenoesophageal ligament and crura are dissected next. The Penrose drain placed during the thoracic phase of the operation can be retrieved, used to retract the gastroesophageal junction, and assist the dissection at the hiatus. It is sometimes necessary to complete the hiatal dissection before dividing the left gastric artery to facilitate passage of the stapler around the vessel with tips of the stapler passing through the hiatus.

The gastric tube is then created with sequential firings of a heavy tissue linear endoscopic stapler (**Fig. 3**). It can be helpful to perform on-table endoscopy to ensure an adequate distal margin. The gastric tube is fashioned by starting the division of the stomach from the lesser curve and dividing toward the fundus. Strong consideration should be given to insertion of a feeding jejunostomy and pyloric drainage procedure.

Delivery of the Specimen and Reconstruction Phase

Several options exist for removal of the specimen and reconstruction of the alimentary tract. If an Ivor-Lewis MIE approach is used, the abdominal phase proceeds to the

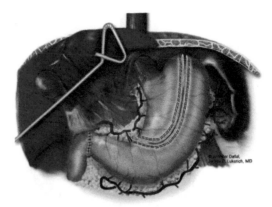

Fig. 3. Creation of a gastric tube. (*Courtesy of* James Luketich, MD, Pittsburgh, PA. Copyright © Jennifer Dallal, MD and James Luketich, MD.)

thoracic phase of the operation. After division of the stomach and creation of the gastric tube, the tip of the conduit is sutured to the distal edge of the specimen margin, taking care to avoid torsion of the conduit. It is important to make sure the hiatus is adequately opened during the laparoscopic dissection to allow passage of the conduit. During the thoracic phase of the operation, the esophagus is transected high in the thorax and the specimen is delivered through an enlarged thoracic port. As the esophagus is delivered out of the chest, the conduit will follow up from the abdomen. The anastomosis can then be created, most commonly performed with a circular end-to-end anastomosis stapler.

If a cervical anastomosis is preferred, the dissection occurs in the right thoracic cavity first, followed by a simultaneous abdominal and cervical dissection. Once the stomach is divided and the tip of the conduit sutured to the distal staple line, the specimen can be delivered by pulling the specimen up through a left cervical incision after transection of the cervical esophagus. Alternatively, a "hybrid" approach can be performed with a small upper midline incision created to remove the specimen from the abdomen after transection of the cervical esophagus. If the stomach is well mobilized, this latter technique allows for delivery of the esophagus and the majority of the stomach out of the abdomen for extracorporeal creation of the gastric conduit and oversewing the staple line if desired. The gastric conduit is passed through to the neck attached to a chest tube or Foley catheter, and the cervical anastomosis can be performed in a hand-sewn or stapled fashion.

OUTCOME OF MINIMALLY INVASIVE ESOPHAGECTOMY

Unlike other minimally invasive operations, the adoption of MIE has been slow and has not supplanted open esophagectomy as the operation of choice. Potentially this is due to the inherent morbidity and mortality associated with esophagectomy, lack of a universally accepted open or minimally invasive surgical approach, a steep learning curve for the minimally invasive operation, and an unclear benefit over open surgery. A handful of centers around the world have pioneered this operation and have reported their results; however, few comparative or randomized trials to assess the benefits of MIE in comparison with open esophagectomy have been performed **(Table 1)**.

Table 1					
Results from select series of open and minimally invasive esophagectomy					
Authors,[Ref.] Year	Technique	No. of Patients	30-Day Mortality (%)	Respiratory Complications (%)	No. of Lymph Nodes
Luketich et al,[17] 2003	MIE (TT)	222	1	20.3	NR
Luketich et al,[22] 2012	MIE (TT + IL)	1011	1.7	NR	21
Biere et al,[16] 2012	MIE (TT)	59	2	12	20
	Open (TT)	56	0	34	21
Mamidanna et al,[6] 2012	MIE	1155	4.0	19.0	NR
	Open	6347	4.3	18.6	
Braghetto et al,[30] 2006	MIE	47	6	15	NR
	Open (TT)	60	12	20	
	Open (TH)	59	10	17	
Orringer et al,[31] 2007	Open (TH)	2007	3	NR	NR
Hulscher et al,[19] 2002	Open (TT)	114	4	57	31
	Open (TH)	106	2	27	16

Abbreviations: IL, Ivor-Lewis esophagectomy; MIE, minimally invasive esophagectomy; NR, not reported; TH, transhiatal esophagectomy; TT, transthoracic esophagectomy.

Early (In-Hospital) Outcomes

Complications following open esophageal resection are common. Similarly, morbidity following MIE remains high. Luketich and colleagues,[17] in a series of 222 patients, reported a major morbidity rate of 32% following MIE. A recent national administrative database analysis from the United Kingdom studied 1155 MIE patients compared with 6347 open esophagectomies over the same time period, and found the morbidity following MIE was 38.0% compared with 39.2% for open esophagectomy ($P = .457$).[6] Some studies have demonstrated improvement in morbidity rates following MIE. Schoppmann and colleagues[18] reported a single-center, case-controlled study comparing MIE with open esophagectomy in 62 patients matched for tumor stage and location, age, sex, and American Society of Anesthesiologists score, overall morbidity was 25% for patients following MIE compared with 74% following open esophagectomy.

Pulmonary complications represent a significant challenge following esophagectomy and account for a significant proportion of total morbidity. A recent randomized controlled trial of open transthoracic versus open transhiatal esophagectomy reported the incidence of pulmonary complications to be 57% and 27%, respectively.[19] Avoidance of a thoracotomy and laparotomy during MIE may result in lower pulmonary complication rates compared with open resection; however, results are mixed. In the only randomized controlled trial of minimally invasive versus open esophagectomy, the incidence of pulmonary infections was significantly lower in the MIE group (12% vs 34%, $P = .005$).[16] Similarly, in the single-center case-controlled series of matched patients, the prevalence of respiratory complications was significantly less in the MIE group (9.7% vs 38.7%, $P = .008$) resulting in a shorter hospital stays and time in the intensive care unit.[18] Another study from Australia comparing 858 patients found MIE to be protective against respiratory failure (odds ratio [OR] 0.11, $P > .001$); however, MIE provided no benefit against pneumonia (OR 1.20, $P = .270$).[20] The review of the United Kingdom's national administrative database found pulmonary complication were similar in both open esophagectomy and MIE. Specifically, there was no difference between the 2 groups in the incidence of pneumonia (19.9% vs 18.6%) or respiratory failure (4.0% vs 3.7%).[6]

The major Achilles heel following esophagectomy remains anastomotic complications. Anastomotic leak rates in recent reports for MIE range from 0% to 33%.[1] In the Pittsburgh series, Luketich and colleagues[17] report a leak rate of 11.7%. By comparison, the leak rate in the randomized controlled trial of open esophagectomy was 15%.[19] The randomized controlled trial of minimally invasive versus open esophagectomy showed no difference in leak rate (MIE 7% vs open 12%; $P = .390$), although the study was not powered to detect a difference in anastomotic leak rates.[16]

Much has been written about mortality following open esophagectomy. Birkmeyer and colleagues[14,21] identified low-volume hospitals (mortality 23%) and low-volume surgeons (mortality = 19%) as important risk factors for mortality following esophagectomy. In experienced centers with experienced surgeons, however, mortality following open esophagectomy is less than 5%.[19] Reported mortality following MIE is similarly low in experienced hands. In the follow-up study of their first 1000 MIEs, the University of Pittsburgh group reports a hospital mortality following MIE of only 2.8%.[22] Others have reported mortality varying between 0% and 6%, which compares favorably with open resection.[1] The recent analysis of the United Kingdom national administrative database study found no difference in 30-day mortality (MIE 4.0% vs open 4.3%; $P = .65$).[6] Similarly, the randomized controlled trial from Europe had similar in-hospital mortality for both groups (MIE 3%, open 2%).[16]

Although the incidence of complications following MIE in these reports may reflect the learning curve of these select surgeons, potential patient selection, or publication bias, the morbidity and mortality following minimally invasive esophagectomy is at least comparable with open esophagectomy. There appears to be a benefit in the incidence of pulmonary complications, but this is not seen across all studies. The development of complications following either open esophagectomy or MIE may have less to do with the incisions but may reflect the complexity and physiologic impact of an esophagectomy.

Oncologic Outcome

The ideal treatment approach to maximize oncologic outcome following resection for esophageal cancer is controversial. Though previously contested, neoadjuvant chemoradiotherapy has gained significant support and is recommended for most patients except those with early-stage disease.[23] Debate, however, continues over the optimal surgical approach, and has centered on the benefits of a transthoracic lymphadenectomy over a simple transhiatal esophagectomy and the extent of lymphadenectomy. A randomized controlled trial of open transthoracic resection versus open transhiatal esophagectomy found a 5-year survival benefit of 39% versus 29%, although this did not achieve statistical significance.[19] However, the study was designed with an estimated 50% benefit in survival at 2 years between the 2 groups, and therefore may have been underpowered to detect the smaller difference. A later subgroup analysis from this trial found that patients with limited nodal disease had a significant 5-year survival benefit (64% vs 23%, $P = .02$) following transthoracic resection.[24] In addition, there is increasing evidence that a more extensive lymphadenectomy is associated with improved survival.[25,26]

As MIE becomes more common, the oncologic impact of a minimally invasive approach to resection must be scrutinized. Unfortunately, there are few data examining the oncologic outcome of MIE versus open surgery. Case series of MIE report lymph node harvests of 5 to 23 lymph nodes.[1] ECOG 2202, a multicenter trial to assess the feasibility of MIE, had a median lymph node harvest of 20 lymph nodes.[27]

Biere and colleagues[16] found a similar number of lymph nodes resected between the open (21, range 7–47) and MIE (20, range 3–44) groups ($P = .852$). Few data exist regarding the locoregional recurrence rate, besides the ECOG 2202 trial reporting a locoregional recurrence rate of 6.7% at 3 years.[27] It seems that an adequate lymphadenectomy can be performed minimally invasively but that long-term survival studies are needed to assess the oncologic impact of MIE.

Quality of Life

Although its impact on morbidity and cancer survival is unclear, MIE does appear to have improved the quality of life when compared with open esophagectomy. At short-term 6-week follow-up, Biere and colleagues[16] found that patients who underwent MIE had significantly improved quality of life as measured by the Short-Form 36 and the European Organization for Research and Treatment of Cancer (EORTC) quality-of-life questionnaires. Sundaram and colleagues,[28] in a single-center experience, compared a small cohort of patients following open transthoracic, open transhiatal, and minimally invasive esophagectomy using the EORTC Quality-of-Life instrument. Patients following MIE reported higher quality of life in nearly all categories of the esophageal cancer quality-of-life module. Pennathur and colleagues[29] reported that of their cohort of 47 patients following MIE for early-stage cancer, 89% of patients had excellent quality of life using the Gastroesophageal Reflux Disease Health-Related Quality-of-Life instrument. In a separate study from the same center, a cohort of 57 patients examined presurgery and postsurgery with the Short-Form 36 questionnaire had excellent preservation of quality of life after MIE.[17]

SUMMARY

Esophagectomy is a complex operation with a significant risk of morbidity and mortality whether performed open or minimally invasively. MIE has a reduced incidence of pulmonary complications and improved quality of life, with a comparable mortality, when performed by experienced esophageal surgeons. A similar harvest of lymph nodes is possible minimally invasively; however, the long-term impact on oncologic outcome remains unanswered and warrants further investigation.

REFERENCES

1. Butler N, Collins S, Memon B, et al. Minimally invasive oesophagectomy: current status and future direction. Surg Endosc 2011;25(7):2071–83.
2. Collard JM, Lengele B, Otte JB, et al. En bloc and standard esophagectomies by thoracoscopy. Ann Thorac Surg 1993;56(3):675–9.
3. DePaula AL, Hashiba K, Ferreira EA, et al. Laparoscopic transhiatal esophagectomy with esophagogastroplasty. Surg Laparosc Endosc 1995;5(1):1–5.
4. Nguyen NT, Schauer PR, Luketich JD. Combined laparoscopic and thoracoscopic approach to esophagectomy. J Am Coll Surg 1999;188(3):328–32.
5. Luketich JD, Schauer PR, Christie NA, et al. Minimally invasive esophagectomy. Ann Thorac Surg 2000;70(3):906–11 [discussion: 911–2].
6. Mamidanna R, Bottle A, Aylin P, et al. Short-term outcomes following open versus minimally invasive esophagectomy for cancer in England: a population-based national study. Ann Surg 2012;255(2):197–203.
7. Polk HC Jr, Zeppa R. Hiatal hernia and esophagitis: a survey of indications for operation and technic and results of fundoplication. Ann Surg 1971;173(5):775–81.

8. Dallemagne B, Weerts JM, Jehaes C, et al. Laparoscopic Nissen fundoplication: preliminary report. Surg Laparosc Endosc 1991;1(3):138–43.
9. Kahrilas PJ, Shaheen NJ, Vaezi MF, et al. American Gastroenterological Association Medical Position Statement on the management of gastroesophageal reflux disease. Gastroenterology 2008;135(4):1383–91, 1391.e1–5.
10. Niebisch S, Fleming FJ, Galey KM, et al. Perioperative risk of laparoscopic fundoplication: safer than previously reported—analysis of the American College of Surgeons National Surgical Quality Improvement Program 2005 to 2009. J Am Coll Surg 2012;215(1):61–8.
11. Ackroyd R, Watson DI, Majeed AW, et al. Randomized clinical trial of laparoscopic versus open fundoplication for gastro-oesophageal reflux disease. Br J Surg 2004;91(8):975–82.
12. McKenna RJ Jr, Houck W, Fuller CB. Video-assisted thoracic surgery lobectomy: experience with 1,100 cases. Ann Thorac Surg 2006;81(2):421–5 [discussion: 425–6].
13. Clinical Outcomes of Surgical Therapy Study Group. A comparison of laparoscopically assisted and open colectomy for colon cancer. N Engl J Med 2004; 350(20):2050–9.
14. Birkmeyer JD, Siewers AE, Finlayson EV, et al. Hospital volume and surgical mortality in the United States. N Engl J Med 2002;346(15):1128–37.
15. Suntharalingam M. Definitive chemoradiation in the management of locally advanced esophageal cancer. Semin Radiat Oncol 2007;17(1):22–8.
16. Biere SS, van Berge Henegouwen MI, Maas KW, et al. Minimally invasive versus open oesophagectomy for patients with oesophageal cancer: a multicentre, open-label, randomised controlled trial. Lancet 2012;379(9829):1887–92.
17. Luketich JD, Alvelo-Rivera M, Buenaventura PO, et al. Minimally invasive esophagectomy: outcomes in 222 patients. Ann Surg 2003;238(4):486–94 [discussion: 494–5].
18. Schoppmann SF, Prager G, Langer FB, et al. Open versus minimally invasive esophagectomy: a single-center case controlled study. Surg Endosc 2010; 24(12):3044–53.
19. Hulscher JB, van Sandick JW, de Boer AG, et al. Extended transthoracic resection compared with limited transhiatal resection for adenocarcinoma of the esophagus. N Engl J Med 2002;347(21):1662–9.
20. Zingg U, Smithers BM, Gotley DC, et al. Factors associated with postoperative pulmonary morbidity after esophagectomy for cancer. Ann Surg Oncol 2011; 18(5):1460–8.
21. Birkmeyer JD, Stukel TA, Siewers AE, et al. Surgeon volume and operative mortality in the United States. N Engl J Med 2003;349(22):2117–27.
22. Luketich JD, Pennathur A, Awais O, et al. Outcomes after minimally invasive esophagectomy: review of over 1000 patients. Ann Surg 2012;256(1):95–103.
23. van Hagen P, Hulshof MC, van Lanschot JJ, et al. Preoperative chemoradiotherapy for esophageal or junctional cancer. N Engl J Med 2012;366(22): 2074–84.
24. Omloo JM, Lagarde SM, Hulscher JB, et al. Extended transthoracic resection compared with limited transhiatal resection for adenocarcinoma of the mid/distal esophagus: five-year survival of a randomized clinical trial. Ann Surg 2007; 246(6):992–1000 [discussion: 1000–1].
25. Peyre CG, Hagen JA, DeMeester SR, et al. The number of lymph nodes removed predicts survival in esophageal cancer: an international study on the impact of extent of surgical resection. Ann Surg 2008;248(4):549–56.

26. Hagen JA, DeMeester SR, Peters JH, et al. Curative resection for esophageal adenocarcinoma: analysis of 100 en bloc esophagectomies. Ann Surg 2001; 234(4):520–30 [discussion: 530–1].
27. Luketich JD, Pennathur A, Catalano PJ, et al. Results of a phase II multicenter study of MIE (Eastern Cooperative Oncology Group Study E2202). J Clin Oncol 2009;27:15S [abstract 4516].
28. Sundaram A, Geronimo JC, Willer BL, et al. Survival and quality of life after minimally invasive esophagectomy: a single-surgeon experience. Surg Endosc 2012; 26(1):168–76.
29. Pennathur A, Farkas A, Krasinskas AM, et al. Esophagectomy for T1 esophageal cancer: outcomes in 100 patients and implications for endoscopic therapy. Ann Thorac Surg 2009;87(4):1048–54 [discussion: 1054–5].
30. Braghetto I, Csendes A, Cardemil G, et al. Open transthoracic or transhiatal esophagectomy versus minimally invasive esophagectomy in terms of morbidity, mortality and survival. Surg Endosc 2006;20(11):1681–6.
31. Orringer MB, Marshall B, Chang AC, et al. Two thousand transhiatal esophagectomies: changing trends, lessons learned. Ann Surg 2007;246(3):363–72 [discussion: 372–4].

Video-Assisted Thoracoscopic Surgery Lobectomy for Lung Cancer

Varun Puri, MD*, Bryan F. Meyers, MD, MPH

KEYWORDS

- Lung cancer • Surgery • VATS • Lobectomy

KEY POINTS

- Video-assisted thoracoscopic surgery (VATS) lobectomy is now emerging as the standard of care for resectable early-stage lung cancer.
- VATS lobectomy has equivalent or improved short-and long-term outcomes compared with open approaches.
- VATS lobectomy should be incorporated into thoracic oncologic practices in a stepwise, organized manner.

Videos of 'video assisted thoracoscopic surgery lobectomy' accompany this article at http://www.surgonc.theclinics.com/.

VIDEO-ASSISTED THORACOSCOPIC SURGERY LOBECTOMY-PIONEERING EFFORTS AND FUNDAMENTAL BASIS IN THORACOSCOPY

Thoracoscopic surgery has been a critical advancement in the care of patients with intrathoracic disease. Initially introduced for diagnostic or minor pleural operations, thoracoscopic surgery has a long history. Early pioneers adapted surgical tools used in endoscopy and urologic surgery for thoracoscopy for a variety of conditions, including gunshot wounds; however, the technique was not widely adopted.[1,2] In 1910, a Swedish internist, Jacobaeus, used a trocar and cannula to induce artificial pneumothorax in a female patient with pulmonary tuberculosis.[1] This description popularized thoracoscopy, but little progress was made in its technical applications. Over the next 8 decades, thoracoscopic procedures remained mainly diagnostic or had limited therapeutic application. The 1990s saw major advances in video technology, microcameras, and endoscopic surgical instruments. These technological advances created the perfect milieu for pioneering surgeons to attempt advanced procedures such as lobectomy via a less-invasive thoracoscopic approach.

Department of Surgery, Washington University School of Medicine, 3108 Queeny Tower, Barnes Jewish Hospital Plaza, St Louis, MO 63110, USA
* Corresponding author.
E-mail address: puriv@wudosis.wustl.edu

Surg Oncol Clin N Am 22 (2013) 27–38
http://dx.doi.org/10.1016/j.soc.2012.09.001
1055-3207/13/$ – see front matter © 2013 Elsevier Inc. All rights reserved.

McKenna's[3] report of an initial experience with video-assisted thoracoscopic surgery (VATS) lobectomy in 44 patients in 1994 marked a significant technical advancement in thoracic oncology. In the period immediately after that report, between 1995 and 2000, VATS lobectomy was met with much skepticism, with specific concerns about the technical aspects of the procedure, its oncologic adequacy, and general reluctance in the surgical community to fundamentally change the approach to an operation. To further add to the controversy, and to provide heft to the arguments of the conservatives, 2 different technical approaches were being advocated for dividing the hilar structures, the critical aspect of a lobectomy. McKenna[3] and other authors[4] advocated the individual dissection and division of the pulmonary arteries, pulmonary veins, and the airway. On the other hand, Lewis[5] reported thoracoscopic lobectomy with simultaneous stapling of the vessels and bronchus rather than individual ligation. With this technique, the lobe was initially mobilized with partial completion of the fissure. A linear stapler commonly used for open procedures was then fired across the vessels and bronchus. This procedure created much controversy, because many surgeons viewed this as a large wedge resection, whereas others were concerned about the development of bronchovascular or pulmonary arteriovenous fistulae. This latter technique is rarely performed today, suggesting that the concerns of the detractors of the mass hilar ligation technique were warranted.

Despite these early controversies, some thoracic surgeons saw a clear advantage to the minimally invasive techniques in terms of improved patient comfort and reduction of surgical trauma. By 1997, 23 surgeons had published results of more than 1500 VATS lobectomy operations.[6] These articles mainly focused on the feasibility of the procedure and early results, with some authors reporting 5-year survival comparable to that of conventional open lobectomy.[7]

WIDESPREAD ADOPTION OF VATS (2000–PRESENT)

Over the past decade, VATS lobectomy has evolved from an operation that only a few centers offered to the de facto preferred procedure for early-stage lung cancer. Although 97 papers were published about VATS lobectomy from 1990 to 2000, since 2000 more than 600 reports discussing this operation have been published in PubMed-indexed journals. This transition has been facilitated by 2 factors.

The first factor is the increasing technical comfort of thoracic surgeons with minimally invasive approaches. The use of a utility (minithoracotomy) incision and the associated adaptation of conventional open instruments to VATS operations have enhanced this technical comfort and enabled great strides in the advancement of minimally invasive approaches. The transition and the learning curve have been elegantly described in several reports from academic and private practice settings.[8–10] The authors' practice has seen a significant shift in the approach to patients with early-stage lung cancer. Before 2005, fewer than 15% of lobectomy operations were performed using VATS, whereas by 2009 more than 55% of lobectomies were completed thoracoscopically (**Fig. 1**).

The second major factor that has led to the surge in VATS lobectomy has been the large volume of reports indicating its short-term superiority over and long-term oncologic equivalence to open lobectomy performed via thoracotomy.[11] The general approach of VATS lobectomy has been the focus of a successful cooperative group feasibility study,[12] 3 randomized trials,[13] more than 30 nonrandomized comparative studies,[13] and hundreds of institutional case series. Data from the Society of Thoracic Surgeons (STS) General Thoracic Surgery database for 2006 showed that 32% of

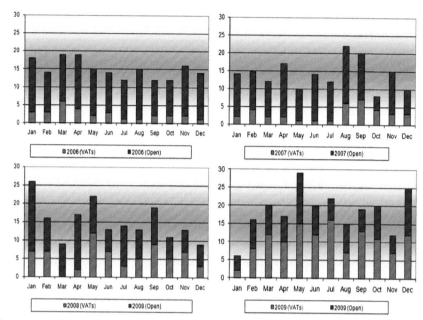

Fig. 1. Relative frequency of VATS and open lobectomy operations at Washington University School of Medicine, St Louis, MO, from 2006 to 2009.

lobectomies for primary lung cancer were performed via VATS,[14] and the proportion is certainly higher now. National thoracic surgical meetings have consistently hosted didactic courses, wet laboratories, and dedicated sessions for VATS lobectomy since 2006, and thoracic surgical residency training programs must ensure adequate exposure to this operation for their trainees to remain competitive.

CURRENT DEFINITION OF VATS LOBECTOMY

Although it is generally agreed that a thoracoscopic lobectomy should be a similar oncologic procedure to an open lobectomy and should imitate established technical principles of that operation, the definition of what constitutes a VATS lobectomy varies greatly. The term can potentially refer to a range of operations, including a standard thoracotomy and lobectomy via a smaller skin incision, or even a giant wedge resection. As an initial step to introduce uniformity to the operation and to study its application in multiple centers, the Cancer and Leukemia Group B (CALGB) 39802 prospective multi-institutional study was designed to elucidate the technical feasibility and safety of VATS in early non–small cell lung cancer (NSCLC) using a standardized definition for VATS lobectomy.[12] The trial defined VATS lobectomy as an operation in which

1. Visualization of intrathoracic structures involves the use of videoscopic equipment (as opposed to direct visualization via a minithoracotomy)
2. No rib spreading occurs
3. Individual dissection of the vein, arteries, and airway is performed for the lobe in question
4. An access incision no longer than 8 cm is created for removal of the lobectomy specimen

5. A standard node sampling or dissection (identical to an open thoracotomy) is performed

Subsequently, multiple authors have described technical variations of this outline, but this general definition of VATS lobectomy has found widespread acceptance. Some of the more common technical nuances within the broad definition of VATS lobectomy are summarized in **Table 1**.

OUTCOMES
Intraoperative Issues

Bleeding from a major pulmonary vessel during VATS can be dangerous because of the limited access. However, because of the lower-pressure pulmonary vascular system, hemorrhage can nearly always be controlled through application of gentle pressure with a broad sponge stick. With the bleeding temporarily controlled, a decision is made as to whether the bleeding can be definitively controlled with VATS or a thoracotomy is needed. Even in the early experience, the incidence of major intraoperative bleeding was low. A collective report by McKenna[6] from 2000 noted that bleeding led to the conversion to a thoracotomy in 10 of 1120 cases from 8 institutions (0.9%). No deaths resulted from the bleeding episodes, and not all patients required transfusion. Over the past decade, numerous reports have described a 0% to 5% conversion rate to thoracotomy because of intraoperative bleeding. In comparative reports, the average blood loss of VATS and open lobectomy have been similar and generally less than 250 mL.[15] Although publication bias may lead to an underappreciation of the incidence and severity of this problem, it seems to be a manageable and generally preventable problem.

Postoperative Outcomes

Most papers comparing VATS with open lobectomy are retrospective single-institutional series and collective reports. Nevertheless, a general clear trend has been seen toward fewer perioperative complications with the VATS approach.[11] These range from fewer postoperative arrhythmias to lower incidence of pneumonia and other respiratory complications. The perioperative mortality for VATS lobectomy is comparable to open surgery. The length of chest tube drainage and hospital stay is reduced with VATS lobectomy. A summary of these reports is presented in **Table 2**.

Table 1 Technical variations in VATS lobectomy	
Technique	**Comment**
Position	Lateral decubitus with or without table flexion, Some use slight posterior tilt
Number of incisions	2–4
Intrathoracic access	Direct or via thoracoscopic/laparoscopic ports
Carbon dioxide insufflation	Occasionally used
Videoscope	0° or 30°
Instruments	Standard thoracotomy set or laparoscopic instruments
Division of vasculature	Stapled, ties, or energy device
Lymph nodes	Complete dissection or systematic sampling

Table 2						
A summary of short-term outcomes after VATS lobectomy						
Author, Year	Type of Report	Approach	Number of Patients	Complications (%)	Length of Hospitalization (d)	Mortality
Kirby et al,[16] 1995	Prospective	VATS	25	24	7.1	0
		Open	30	53	8.3	0
Petersen et al,[17] 2007	Retrospective	VATS	43	27	4	0
		Open	57	35	5	0
Whitson et al,[18] 2007	Retrospective	VATS	59	Pneumonia: 3	6.4	0
		Open	88	19	7.7	0
Whitson et al,[11] 2008	Review	VATS	3114	16.4	8.3	NR
		Open	3256	31.2	13.3	NR
Villamizar et al,[19] 2009	Retrospective	VATS	284	31	4	3
		Open	284	49	5	5
Flores et al,[20] 2009	Retrospective	VATS	398	24	5	0.3
		Open	343	30	7	0.3
Yan et al,[21] 2009	Review	VATS	1391	NR	12	0.4
		Open	1250	NR	12.2	0.7
Scott et al,[22] 2010	Prospective	VATS	66	27	5	0
		Open	686	48	7	1.6
Park et al,[23] 2012	Retrospective	VATS	1523	38	5	1.5
		Open	4769	44	7	2.2

Abbreviation: NR, not reported.

Pain Control and Quality of Life

Thoracotomy is one of the most painful surgical procedures, and some patients may also experience postoperative upper extremity dysfunction. Anatomically, the main cause of postoperative pain is direct injury to the chest wall and intercostal nerves. Rib spreading in a thoracotomy can cause uncontrolled rib fractures and impingement of intercostal nerves. The diminished surgical trauma to the chest wall from VATS lobectomy is reflected in diminished levels of postoperative pain.[24–27] The shorter duration of chest tube drainage after VATS lobectomy may also contribute to the lower pain levels. More than 80% of patients still require narcotic analgesics 3 weeks after an open lobectomy compared with fewer than 40% patients after a VATS lobectomy.[28] Reduced pain levels may contribute to the observed improved quality of life (QOL) after a VATS resection.

A 2008 report by Demmy and Nwogu[28] provided a comprehensive review of subjective and objective QOL measures after VATS lobectomy. They reviewed 97 papers and concluded that QOL is improved compared with after open surgery, and this improvement is demonstrated by better scores on standardized QOL instruments, improved physical activity after surgery, and an earlier return to work.[28] Additionally, this relative improvement in QOL and functional status is most marked in older patients (>70 years old), those with emphysema, and those with other significant comorbidities that increase frailty. At discharge, nearly 80% of patients who undergo VATS lobectomy are independent and do not require assistance with activities of daily living or specific nursing care, compared with 30% of those who undergo open lobectomy.[28] Another relevant issue is the ability to tolerate adjuvant chemotherapy when indicated. A report from the Duke thoracic surgery group concluded that patients who undergo VATS lobectomy tolerate postoperative adjuvant therapy significantly better than patients who undergo open lobectomy, showing the superior preservation in performance status afforded by less-invasive surgery.[17]

Long-Term Outcomes

The success of any oncologic procedure can only be truly measured in terms of inter-mediate- to long-term survival compared with the gold standard. Only a few reports presented long-term survival after VATS lobectomy in the 1990s. However, the results were favorable, with McKenna and colleagues[7] reporting a 4.5-year survival of 76% for 212 patients with stage I lung cancer. The growing experience has been reflected in the form of larger series, with the same authors reporting on outcomes from 1100 VATS lobectomy operations in 2006.[29] Of these patients, 497 with stage IA lung cancer had a 5-year survival of 80%. Similar outcomes for VATS lobectomy for stage I lung cancer have now been reported by several other authors, and these are summarized in **Table 3**.

Meanwhile, other authors have compared the long-term survival after VATS versus open lobectomy in several, mainly retrospective, reports. Increasing evidence of comparable long-term survival in nonrandomized comparisons has shown that a large-scale, prospective, randomized trial comparing open and VATS lobectomy is not realistic. It is doubtful that there would be sufficient equipoise to allow VATS enthusiasts to randomize patients to an open approach. **Table 4** summarizes results from reports comparing these 2 approaches.

These reports show an equivalent or slightly improved long-term survival after VATS lobectomy. Given the projected oncologic equivalence of these seemingly identical operations, the potential survival advantage with VATS lobectomy may be hard to explain. The open thoracotomy approach, by virtue of greater surgical trauma, has been hypothesized to be potentially more immunosuppressive than the minimally invasive approach. This global immunosuppression could potentially decrease the patient's ability to scavenge residual tumor cells or cells shed into the bloodstream or lymphatics at the time of resection.

| Table 3 | | | |
| A summary of long-term survival after VATS lobectomy | | | |
Author, Year	Number of Patients	Survival (%)	Follow-Up (y)
Lewis and Caccavale,[30] 1998	400	92	3
Sugi et al,[31] 2000	48	90	5
Kaseda et al,[32] 2000	204	90	5
Solaini et al,[27] 2001	125	90	3
Walker et al,[25] 2003	158	78	5
Iwasaki et al,[33] 2004	100	78	5
Ohtuska et al,[34] 2004	106	93	3
Roviaro et al,[26] 2004	257	64	5
Kim et al,[35] 2010	704	95	3

Table 4
Comparative studies of VATS and open lobectomy: long-term results

Author, Year	Type of Study	Clinical Stage	Patients (n)	Follow-Up/ Duration of Analysis (y)	Survival With VATS (%)	Survival With Open (%)
Sugi et al,[36] 2000	Prospective, randomized	I	VATS: 48 Open: 52	5	90	85
Shiraishi et al,[37] 2006	Retrospective	I	VATS: 81 Open: 79	5	89	78
Whitson et al,[11] 2008	Review	I/II	VATS: 3114 Open: 3256	5	80	66
Flores et al,[20] 2009	Retrospective	I	VATS: 398 Open: 43	5	79	75
Yang et al,[38] 2009	Retrospective	I	VATS: 113 Open: 508	5	79 (Stage I)	82 (Stage I)
Farjah et al,[39] 2009	Retrospective (SEER data)	Variable	VATS: 721 Open: 12237	NR	VATS vs open: hazard ratio, 0.97	

Abbreviation: Surveillance, Epidemiology and End Results Program.

TECHNIQUE

Several authors have described the technical aspects of VATS lobectomy.[6,40] The following videos illustrate the authors' technique for VATS lobectomy (Videos 1–4).

CONTROVERSIES
Learning Curve

The numerous publications on VATS lobectomy suggest that the thoracic surgical community had ascended the learning curve for this operation by 2005, but individual surgeons and centers have continued to learn and refine the operation. Belgers and colleagues[10] described their learning curve and elucidated several common themes and technical points that the authors of this article have also found useful in the early experience. These are:

1. Performing wedge resections and pleural procedures via VATS
2. Having 2 fully trained surgeons scrub for the initial 10 to 20 VATS lobectomies
3. Starting every possible VATS lobectomy thoracoscopically
4. Not viewing a conversion as a failure but as a safety issue
5. Establishing a routine order of dissection for each lobe
6. Paying close attention to the placement of incisions
7. Making the 6- to 8-cm access incision for the initial cases

Ng and Ryder[41] also described the safe transition of a new graduate's practice to VATS lobectomy from an open approach. They used a muscle-sparing thoracotomy as an intermediate step between the 2 approaches. Although no consensus exists on the number of cases required to achieve proficiency at VATS lobectomy, a learning curve ranging from 30 to 50 cases has been described by different authors.[9,41]

However, a general consensus exists in large surveys that VATS lobectomy is an important tool and that every thoracic surgical unit should develop these skills in a graduated manner.[42]

Conversion to Thoracotomy

Conversion from VATS to open thoracotomy is necessary in 0.0% to 19.5% of patients.[6] The conversion rate is widely variable depending on the center, the experience of the surgeon, and the possible willingness to start most pulmonary resections thoracoscopically. McKenna and colleagues[29] reported a low conversion rate of 2.5% in 1100 patients; however, smaller series, especially from programs that are early in the process of adopting this technique, have a higher conversion rate of 5% to 15%.[43] The reasons for conversion are summarized in **Box 1**.

Fortunately, the need to convert rapidly because of bleeding is uncommon. When converting to a thoracotomy, the options are to enlarge the access incision as an axillary thoracotomy or to create a standard posterolateral thoracotomy. The decision is based on the urgency of the situation and the anticipated location in the chest where exposure is most needed. A controlled planned conversion is usually not a major disruption to the patient's perioperative course. Perioperative pain control should be addressed with subpleural local anesthetic infusion systems or epidural catheters in these patients. Again, one must view orderly and methodical conversions as adherence to a safety policy rather than as a technical shortcoming.

Robotic Lobectomy

The application of robotic technology to anatomic pulmonary resections is a recent development. This practice has been a polarizing issue in thoracic surgery, with strong opinions and arguments on both sides of the issue. Robotic lobectomy has been shown to be safe and effective, providing improved perioperative outcomes and equivalent oncologic results compared with open lobectomy via thoracotomy.[44–46] Not much doubt exists that robotic lobectomy provides all the advantages of a minimally invasive operation. When compared with VATS lobectomy, proponents of robotic lobectomy cite the improved visualization of the field, better wrist-like motion of the instruments, and possibly an easier technical transition from open to robotic lobectomy rather than to VATS lobectomy. Proponents of VATS lobectomy cite the lack of any foreseeable advantage over VATS, an already well-proven technique,

---

Box 1
Common reasons for conversion of VATS to open lobectomy

Oncologic

    Large tumors (often >6–7 cm)

    Unanticipated need for sleeve resection

    Tumor adherence to chest wall/diaphragm/mediastinum

Other technical

    Adherent hilar nodes (malignant/granulomatous)

    Bleeding from hilar vessels

    Pleural adhesions

    Failure to progress at reasonable pace

and the substantial additional costs associated with robotic technology.[47] Additionally, the safety and efficacy of VATS for hilar and lymph node dissection has been established over more than 2 decades. Meanwhile, the possible incorporation of better camera technology and wristed operating instruments as direct maneuvers may strengthen the case for VATS lobectomy. No direct comparative reports of VATS versus robotic lobectomy have been published to date. As more data become available, the debate is likely to continue for the foreseeable future. Additional technological advances in either practice may play a role in this debate.

Reimbursement Issues

Although reimbursement for providers for medical procedures varies with the type of insurance, Medicare current procedural terminology (CPT) codes are a well-accepted way to compare procedures. An open lobectomy (CPT 32480) with mediastinal lymph node dissection (CPT 38746) generates 51.35 total RVUs (relative value units), whereas a VATS lobectomy (CPT 32663) with mediastinal lymph node dissection (CPT 32674) generates 48.75 total RVUs. It is mildly surprising to note that the provider compensation for VATS is lower, given the additional technical skill involved and the likelihood that extra provider effort has been invested in learning new techniques. In addition to patient benefits over an open approach, a higher level of coding would be an added incentive to learn and apply new skills. The codes for robotic lobectomy are identical to those for VATS lobectomy.

Immunologic Issues

Changes in the immune system after surgery for cancer may provide information relevant to the short-term and long-term patient survival. The effect of VATS lobectomy on the inflammatory/immune system has been studied by several authors.[36,48–50] Early studies showed that the VATS approach is associated with less tissue and vascular trauma, and consequently reduces the activity of acute phase cytokines and their receptors (interleukin 6, tumor necrosis factor) and inflammatory mediators (C-reactive protein) in the perioperative period.[49] The theory is that patients undergoing open lobectomy for NSCLC experience a greater degree of surgical stress that may inhibit their baseline immune function, leaving them susceptible to infectious complications or to lessened tumor surveillance, thus potentially diminishing survival.[48] Analysis of peripheral blood mononuclear cells has shown that VATS lobectomy for NSCLC is associated with less impairment of cellular cytotoxicity compared with thoracotomy.[48] Although these immunologic data are enticing, they currently do not offer conclusive proof of the purported oncologic advantage of VATS lobectomy.

SUMMARY

VATS lobectomy is a safe and feasible operation for early-stage lung cancer. The transition from open to VATS approach can be safely made in academic and practice settings. VATS lobectomy improves short-term patient-centered outcomes compared with an open approach and is at least equivalent to the open approach in long-term oncologic outcomes and survival. VATS lobectomy should be considered the preferred operation for early-stage lung cancer.

SUPPLEMENTARY DATA

Supplementary data related to this article can be found online at http://dx.doi.org/10.1016/j.soc.2012.09.001.

REFERENCES

1. Hoksch B, Birken-Bertsch H, Muller JM. Thoracoscopy before Jacobaeus. Ann Thorac Surg 2002;74:1288–90.
2. Solli P, Spaggiari L. Indications and developments of video-assisted thoracic surgery in the treatment of lung cancer. Oncologist 2007;12:1205–14.
3. McKenna RJ Jr. Lobectomy by video-assisted thoracic surgery with mediastinal node sampling for lung cancer. J Thorac Cardiovasc Surg 1994;107:879–81 [discussion: 881–72].
4. Hermansson U, Konstantinov IE, Aren C. Video-assisted thoracic surgery (VATS) lobectomy: the initial Swedish experience. Semin Thorac Cardiovasc Surg 1998; 10:285–90.
5. Lewis RJ. The role of video-assisted thoracic surgery for carcinoma of the lung: wedge resection to lobectomy by simultaneous individual stapling. Ann Thorac Surg 1993;56:762–8.
6. McKenna RJ Jr. Thoracoscopic evaluation and treatment of pulmonary disease. Surg Clin North Am 2000;80:1543–53.
7. McKenna RJ Jr, Fischel RJ, Wolf R, et al. Video-assisted thoracic surgery (VATS) lobectomy for bronchogenic carcinoma. Semin Thorac Cardiovasc Surg 1998;10:321–5.
8. Zhao H, Bu L, Yang F, et al. Video-assisted thoracoscopic surgery lobectomy for lung cancer: the learning curve. World J Surg 2010;34:2368–72.
9. Petersen RH, Hansen HJ. Learning thoracoscopic lobectomy. Eur J Cardiothorac Surg 2010;37:516–20.
10. Belgers EH, Siebenga J, Bosch AM, et al. Complete video-assisted thoracoscopic surgery lobectomy and its learning curve. A single center study introducing the technique in The Netherlands. Interact Cardiovasc Thorac Surg 2010;10:176–80.
11. Whitson BA, Groth SS, Duval SJ, et al. Surgery for early-stage non-small cell lung cancer: a systematic review of the video-assisted thoracoscopic surgery versus thoracotomy approaches to lobectomy. Ann Thorac Surg 2008;86:2008–16 [discussion: 2016–8].
12. Swanson SJ, Herndon JE 2nd, D'Amico TA, et al. Video-assisted thoracic surgery lobectomy: report of CALGB 39802–a prospective, multi-institution feasibility study. J Clin Oncol 2007;25:4993–7.
13. Cheng D, Downey RJ, Kernstine K, et al. Video-assisted thoracic surgery in lung cancer resection: a meta-analysis and systematic review of controlled trials. Innovations (Phila) 2007;2:261–92.
14. Boffa DJ, Allen MS, Grab JD, et al. Data from the society of thoracic surgeons general thoracic surgery database: the surgical management of primary lung tumors. J Thorac Cardiovasc Surg 2008;135:247–54.
15. Gorenstein LA, Sonett JR. The surgical management of stage I and stage II lung cancer. Surg Oncol Clin N Am 2011;20:701–20.
16. Kirby TJ, Mack MJ, Landreneau RJ, et al. Lobectomy–video-assisted thoracic surgery versus muscle-sparing thoracotomy. A randomized trial. J Thorac Cardiovasc Surg 1995;109:997–1001 [discussion: 1001–2].
17. Petersen RP, Pham D, Burfeind WR, et al. Thoracoscopic lobectomy facilitates the delivery of chemotherapy after resection for lung cancer. Ann Thorac Surg 2007; 83:1245–9 [discussion: 1250].
18. Whitson BA, Andrade RS, Boettcher A, et al. Video-assisted thoracoscopic surgery is more favorable than thoracotomy for resection of clinical stage I non-small cell lung cancer. Ann Thorac Surg 2007;83:1965–70.

19. Villamizar NR, Darrabie MD, Burfeind WR, et al. Thoracoscopic lobectomy is associated with lower morbidity compared with thoracotomy. J Thorac Cardiovasc Surg 2009;138:419–25.

20. Flores RM, Park BJ, Dycoco J, et al. Lobectomy by video-assisted thoracic surgery (VATS) versus thoracotomy for lung cancer. J Thorac Cardiovasc Surg 2009;138:11–8.

21. Yan TD, Black D, Bannon PG, et al. Systematic review and meta-analysis of randomized and nonrandomized trials on safety and efficacy of video-assisted thoracic surgery lobectomy for early-stage non-small-cell lung cancer. J Clin Oncol 2009;27:2553–62.

22. Scott WJ, Allen MS, Darling G, et al. Video-assisted thoracic surgery versus open lobectomy for lung cancer: a secondary analysis of data from the American College of Surgeons Oncology Group Z0030 randomized clinical trial. J Thorac Cardiovasc Surg 2010;139:976–81 [discussion: 981–73].

23. Park HS, Detterbeck FC, Boffa DJ, et al. Impact of hospital volume of thoracoscopic lobectomy on primary lung cancer outcomes. Ann Thorac Surg 2012; 93:372–9.

24. Daniels LJ, Balderson SS, Onaitis MW, et al. Thoracoscopic lobectomy: a safe and effective strategy for patients with stage I lung cancer. Ann Thorac Surg 2002;74:860–4.

25. Walker WS, Codispoti M, Soon SY, et al. Long-term outcomes following VATS lobectomy for non-small cell bronchogenic carcinoma. Eur J Cardiothorac Surg 2003;23:397–402.

26. Roviaro G, Varoli F, Vergani C, et al. Long-term survival after videothoracoscopic lobectomy for stage I lung cancer. Chest 2004;126:725–32.

27. Solaini L, Prusciano F, Bagioni P, et al. Video-assisted thoracic surgery major pulmonary resections. Present experience. Eur J Cardiothorac Surg 2001;20:437–42.

28. Demmy TL, Nwogu C. Is video-assisted thoracic surgery lobectomy better? Quality of life considerations. Ann Thorac Surg 2008;85:S719–28.

29. McKenna RJ Jr, Houck W, Fuller CB. Video-assisted thoracic surgery lobectomy: experience with 1,100 cases. Ann Thorac Surg 2006;81:421–5 [discussion: 425–6].

30. Lewis RJ, Caccavale RJ. Video-assisted thoracic surgical non-rib spreading simultaneously stapled lobectomy (VATS(n)SSL). Semin Thorac Cardiovasc Surg 1998;10:332–9.

31. Sugi K, Kaneda Y, Esato K. Video-assisted thoracoscopic lobectomy achieves a satisfactory long-term prognosis in patients with clinical stage IA lung cancer. World J Surg 2000;24:27–30 [discussion: 30–21].

32. Kaseda S, Aoki T, Hangai N, et al. Better pulmonary function and prognosis with video-assisted thoracic surgery than with thoracotomy. Ann Thorac Surg 2000;70: 1644–6.

33. Iwasaki A, Shirakusa T, Shiraishi T, et al. Results of video-assisted thoracic surgery for stage I/II non-small cell lung cancer. Eur J Cardiothorac Surg 2004; 26:158–64.

34. Ohtsuka T, Nomori H, Horio H, et al. Is major pulmonary resection by video-assisted thoracic surgery an adequate procedure in clinical stage I lung cancer? Chest 2004;125:1742–6.

35. Kim K, Kim HK, Park JS, et al. Video-assisted thoracic surgery lobectomy: single institutional experience with 704 cases. Ann Thorac Surg 2010;89:S2118–22.

36. Sugi K, Kaneda Y, Esato K. Video-assisted thoracoscopic lobectomy reduces cytokine production more than conventional open lobectomy. Jpn J Thorac Cardiovasc Surg 2000;48:161–5.

37. Shiraishi T, Shirakusa T, Hiratsuka M, et al. Video-assisted thoracoscopic surgery lobectomy for c-T1N0M0 primary lung cancer: its impact on locoregional control. Ann Thorac Surg 2006;82:1021–6.
38. Yang X, Qu J, Wang S. Long-term outcomes of video-assisted thoracic surgery lobectomy for nonsmall cell lung cancer. South Med J 2009;102:905–8.
39. Farjah F, Wood DE, Mulligan MS, et al. Safety and efficacy of video-assisted versus conventional lung resection for lung cancer. J Thorac Cardiovasc Surg 2009;137:1415–21.
40. Demmy TL, James TA, Swanson SJ, et al. Troubleshooting video-assisted thoracic surgery lobectomy. Ann Thorac Surg 2005;79:1744–52 [discussion: 1753].
41. Ng T, Ryder BA. Evolution to video-assisted thoracic surgery lobectomy after training: initial results of the first 30 patients. J Am Coll Surg 2006;203:551–7.
42. Rocco G, Internullo E, Cassivi SD, et al. The variability of practice in minimally invasive thoracic surgery for pulmonary resections. Thorac Surg Clin 2008;18: 235–47.
43. Zhu M, Fu XN, Chen X. Lobectomy by video-assisted thoracoscopic surgery (VATS) for early stage of non-small cell lung cancer. Front Med 2011;5:53–60.
44. Cerfolio RJ, Bryant AS, Skylizard L, et al. Initial consecutive experience of completely portal robotic pulmonary resection with 4 arms. J Thorac Cardiovasc Surg 2011;142:740–6.
45. Park BJ, Melfi F, Mussi A, et al. Robotic lobectomy for non-small cell lung cancer (NSCLC): long-term oncologic results. J Thorac Cardiovasc Surg 2012;143: 383–9.
46. Park BJ, Flores RM, Rusch VW. Robotic assistance for video-assisted thoracic surgical lobectomy: technique and initial results. J Thorac Cardiovasc Surg 2006;131:54–9.
47. Swanson SJ. Robotic pulmonary lobectomy–the future and probably should remain so. J Thorac Cardiovasc Surg 2010;140:954.
48. Whitson BA, D'Cunha J, Andrade RS, et al. Thoracoscopic versus thoracotomy approaches to lobectomy: differential impairment of cellular immunity. Ann Thorac Surg 2008;86:1735–44.
49. Craig SR, Leaver HA, Yap PL, et al. Acute phase responses following minimal access and conventional thoracic surgery. Eur J Cardiothorac Surg 2001;20: 455–63.
50. Yim AP, Wan S, Lee TW, et al. VATS lobectomy reduces cytokine responses compared with conventional surgery. Ann Thorac Surg 2000;70:243–7.

Laparoscopic Gastrectomy for Cancer

Joseph D. Phillips, MD[a], Alexander P. Nagle, MD[b,*],
Nathaniel J. Soper, MD[a]

KEYWORDS

- Gastric cancer • Laparoscopic gastrectomy • Gastric carcinoma
- Minimally invasive gastrectomy

KEY POINTS

- Differences between Eastern and Western countries exist in both location and stage of gastric cancer at presentation. In addition, patients in the West tend to be, on average, older, have a higher BMI, and have more extensive comorbidities.
- Staging laparoscopy is done with adjunct studies such as peritoneal cytology and intraoperative ultrasound, which are valuable tools in the diagnostic evaluation of patients with potentially resectable disease.
- Laparoscopic gastrectomy is a challenging operation; advanced laparoscopic skills are required to perform an adequate lymphadenectomy and an intestinal anastomosis in an oncologically appropriate manner.
- Numerous studies from Asia have demonstrated the benefits of laparoscopic gastrectomy for malignancy while maintaining equivalent short-term and long-term oncologic outcomes compared with open surgery. In the United States, further experience and standardization are needed before these techniques will become widely accepted.
- As surgeons continue to investigate minimally invasive techniques for gastric cancer, new technologies may be developed that shorten the extensive learning curve required to master these complex procedures.

INTRODUCTION

Laparoscopic gastrectomy for gastric cancer was pioneered in Eastern Asia, where the incidence of gastric cancer is high and population-based screening programs exist. In 1994, Kitano and colleagues[1] performed the first laparoscopic-assisted distal

Disclosures: All authors have nothing to disclose.
[a] Department of Surgery, Feinberg School of Medicine, Northwestern University, East Huron Street, Galter 3-150, Chicago, IL 60611, USA; [b] Department of Surgery, Feinberg School of Medicine, Northwestern University, 676 North Street Clair Avenue, Suite 6-650, Chicago, IL 60611, USA
* Corresponding author.
E-mail address: anagle@nmh.org

gastrectomy with lymph node dissection for gastric cancer. Since that time there has been a plethora of data from eastern Asia demonstrating the safety, feasibly, and oncologic outcomes of laparoscopic gastrectomy. In Western countries, Belgium and Italy have been on the forefront of advancing laparoscopic gastrectomy for malignancy. In 1993, Azagra and colleagues[2,3] performed the first laparoscopic distal gastrectomy with Billroth II anastomosis for gastric cancer and, in 1995, this group reported the first laparoscopic total gastrectomy for cancer. Huscher and colleagues,[4] from Italy, reported the only prospective, randomized trial to date in the West regarding 5-year clinical outcomes of laparoscopic-assisted subtotal gastrectomy compared with open surgery for stage-matched adenocarcinomas, demonstrating both safety and feasibility of the laparoscopic approach. Five-year survival numbers showed no significant difference between the two groups, but patients in the laparoscopic group had less blood loss, earlier oral intake and shorter hospital stay.

In the United States, the role of laparoscopy for the treatment of cancer has evolved considerably, but at a much slower pace. The short-term benefits of laparoscopy compared with laparotomy are apparent, but the main concerns have centered on oncologic equivalency. Specifically, these issues include recurrence and survival, the ability to laparoscopically obtain negative margins and perform an adequate lymph node dissection, the potential for local tumor dissemination and port-site metastasis, and the effects of CO_2 pneumoperitoneum. As these issues have been addressed by studies in support of laparoscopic surgery for colorectal cancer, the use of laparoscopy for malignancy has increased.[5,6] However, in the United States, there are few data regarding the role of laparoscopic gastrectomy in the treatment of gastric carcinoma. Literature from the United States contains only five retrospective comparative studies, with the largest report including only 30 patients in the laparoscopic group. This may be related to the lower incidence of gastric cancer in the United States and the higher proportion of locally advanced disease at diagnosis.[7] In addition, there is a significant learning curve for these advanced laparoscopic procedures. As such, in the United States, the use of laparoscopic gastrectomy for the treatment of gastric cancer is low and remains somewhat controversial. However, as investigation of advanced laparoscopy for gastric cancer continues and results of randomized trials become available, surgeons will gain more experience and techniques will become more standardized and broadly accepted. Currently laparoscopic gastrectomy for gastric cancer should be considered only in select cases. Patients with early mucosal disease seem to be good candidates for a laparoscopic approach given the low (<3%) risk of nodal disease.[8] In addition, patients with advanced disease may be suitable candidates for a laparoscopic palliative resection. However, for most patients in the United States who present with locally advanced disease, laparoscopic gastrectomy should be recommended only within the confines of investigational trials at centers experienced in treating patients with gastric cancer.

EPIDEMIOLOGY

Gastric cancer is the fourth most commonly diagnosed malignancy worldwide, with nearly 990,000 cases per year.[9] Approximately 70% of these cases occur in developing countries. It is the second leading cause of cancer mortality with an estimated 738,000 deaths per year. The highest incidence rates are in Eastern Asian countries, with a male predominance of 2 to 1. In the United States, there are approximately 21,300 cases diagnosed and more than 10,300 deaths yearly.[10] Despite advances in multimodality therapy for gastric cancer, recurrence and mortality remain high. In the United States, the overall 5-year survival for all stages combined is 28%.[10]

Approximately 95% of cases are adenocarcinomas, with the remaining 5% being a mix of lymphoma, carcinoid, leiomyosarcoma, gastrointestinal stromal tumors, adenosquamous, and squamous cell carcinomas.[11]

Differences between Eastern and Western hemisphere countries exist in both location and stage of disease at presentation. In Eastern countries, like Japan and South Korea where much of the data related to laparoscopic gastric surgery originate, cancers tend to be in the middle and distal portions of the stomach. In the West, however, carcinomas of the proximal stomach are increasingly more common. Histologically, intestinal type tumors predominate in the East, while in the West the predominant type is diffuse.[12] In addition, Eastern countries have intense screening programs that detect up to 70% of cancers at an early stage.[13] In contrast, in Western nations most lesions are detected only after causing symptoms such as pain, dysphagia, and anemia, and, as a result, up to 80% of patients will already have advanced disease at diagnosis.[7] Furthermore, patients in the West tend to be an average of 10 years older (average age 70 in the United States), significantly more overweight, have a higher incidence of cardiovascular disease, and a higher risk of thromboembolic complications.[14]

DIAGNOSTIC EVALUATION

Proper staging of patients with gastric cancer is essential for providing the appropriate treatment course and is based on the American Joint Committee on Cancer system, which includes characteristics of the tumor (T), nodal status (N), and metastatic disease (M).[15] A separate Japanese classification system exists[16] but is not as broadly used, especially in the United States. Esophagogastroduodenoscopy and tissue biopsy are essential for pathologic diagnosis. Evaluation should include CT scans of the abdomen and pelvis and, for proximal lesions, CT scan of the chest. Although CT has limited accuracy for assessing the depth of tumor invasion or regional nodal involvement, it may detect distant nodal or visceral metastases, ascites, or carcinomatosis. However, preoperative CT scans often underestimate the extent of disease, principally because of radiographically undetectable metastases involving the liver and peritoneum. Endoscopic ultrasonography (EUS) should also be used to provide a more accurate staging evaluation of the T and N status. EUS has a T-stage accuracy of 60% to 80% and a lymph node accuracy of 50% to 65%. Additionally, EUS allows for fine-needle aspiration of suspicious lymph nodes and can detect liver metastases missed by conventional imaging studies.[17,18] As such, EUS is important in identifying lesions that may be amenable to endoscopic mucosal resection and selecting patients for neoadjuvant therapy. PET scanning may be used as adjunct imaging to detect distant metastases, but approximately 50% of diffuse type tumors are not avid for the principal tracer, fluorodeoxyglucose F 18.[19]

Staging laparoscopy, though more invasive than CT or EUS, has the advantage of directly visualizing the liver surface, peritoneum, and local lymph nodes, and permits biopsy of any suspicious lesions. Furthermore, the stomach can be closely inspected for direct tumor extension into surrounding organs such as the liver, pancreas, colon, and spleen. Bulky nodal disease does not necessarily preclude resection, but lymph nodes outside the planned resection bed or suspicious nodules should be sent for intraoperative frozen section analysis. At laparoscopy, radiologically occult metastases are documented in up to 40% of patients with gastric cancer and a negative CT, who would have been considered potentially resectable. Power and colleagues[20] found that those with T1–2, N0 tumors on EUS were at much lower risk for metastasis at laparoscopy than those with T3–4 or N+ disease (4% vs 25%). In addition, laparoscopic ultrasound is a valuable adjunct to detect and evaluate liver metastases that are not visualized from the surface.[21]

Peritoneal cytology can also be obtained during staging laparoscopy. This is performed by instilling 100 to 200 cc of normal saline into the pouch of Douglas and the paracolic gutters. At least 50 cc should be recovered for cytologic analysis. Patients with peritoneal cytology that is positive for malignant cells (up to 60% of patients with locally advanced disease on imaging) should be treated as having metastatic disease because their survival following resection is similar to those with overt metastases.[22,23] In select cases, patients with positive peritoneal cytology may be reevaluated for resection after chemotherapy, if they demonstrate no evidence of disease progression.[24]

For surgeons who routinely perform open gastrectomy for gastric cancer, the selection of patients who need staging laparoscopy is controversial. Guidelines from the National Comprehensive Cancer Network suggest only that laparoscopy be considered for patients who seem have advanced locoregional disease (T3–4 or N+) after conventional radiographic and EUS staging.[25] The authors' practice is to perform staging laparoscopy with peritoneal cytology for any medically fit patient with locally advanced gastric cancer who does not have histologic confirmation of stage IV disease. Following completion of staging laparoscopy, if the cancer remains resectable with a curative intent, the decision is then made whether to proceed with a laparoscopic gastrectomy or convert to an open procedure.

EARLY GASTRIC CANCER

A thorough understanding of the presentation, natural history, and biologic behavior of gastric cancer, as well as the accurate location and staging of the disease, is critical for providing an oncologically appropriate and safe operation. The extent of surgical resection is determined by the tumor size, depth of invasion, and extent of lymph node involvement. Early gastric cancer (EGC) is defined as a tumor that invades no more than the submucosa (T1). Lesions limited to the mucosa (carcinoma in situ [Tis]–T1a) have a reported rate of regional lymph node metastasis of 1% to 3%, in contrast to lesions that penetrate the submucosa (T1b), which have a rate of 8%–18%, depending on tumor size.[8] Endoscopic mucosal resection and endoscopic submucosal dissection have gained notoriety in Asian countries for patients with EGC and a low risk of lymph node involvement.[17] In Western countries there has been less experience with these techniques, likely owing to the differences in stage at presentation. Current guidelines in the United States limit endoscopic resection to Tis or well to moderately differentiated mucosal lesions (T1a) with no evidence of ulceration, lymphovascular invasion, or lymph node metastases.[25] Alternatively, lesions limited to the mucosa (Tis or T1a) can be resected by laparoscopic wedge resection.[26–28] Preoperative tattooing of the lesion and intraoperative endoscopy are helpful for intraoperative localization. Laparoscopic wedge resection can then be completed with laparoscopic reticulating stapling devices. Careful inspection of the specimen should be made to exclude positive margins. One study reported an 88% 5-year survival, but 26% of patients were found to have submucosal invasion (T1b) on pathologic examination, stressing the importance of accurate preoperative T-staging.[26] Thus, these patients must be followed closely with diligent surveillance for recurrence of disease. T1b lesions are best treated with formal gastric resection. These lesions are well suited for a laparoscopic approach and, in fact, most of the literature regarding laparoscopic gastrectomy for cancer concerns early stage disease.

LOCALLY ADVANCED GASTRIC CANCER

Owing to the increased risk of lymph node involvement and metastatic disease for advanced tumors ($\geq$T3), surgeons were initially cautious with using laparoscopic techniques for advanced gastric cancer. Until recently, investigators recommended against a laparoscopic approach for cancer that was preoperatively staged as more advanced than T2N1.[29,30] However, because so few patients present with EGC in the West, several investigators have recently studied laparoscopic resection for advanced gastric cancer with the hopes of extending the potential benefits of laparoscopy to a larger patient population. The increased complexity and technical difficulty of these operations is related to the greater nodal burden of disease as well as the potential for adherence to surrounding organs, namely the pancreas, spleen, and liver. Initially, there was hesitancy on the part of surgeons to perform these operations laparoscopically without evidence for oncologic equivalency to open procedures. However, as experience with laparoscopic gastric resection has grown, some investigators have begun to expand these techniques to more advanced disease and have demonstrated comparable short-term and long-term outcomes to open resections.[31–34]

EXTENT OF LYMPH NODE DISSECTION

One of the most controversial areas in the surgical management of gastric cancer is the optimal extent of lymph node dissection. Three types of lymph node dissection are performed: perigastric (D1 + α), additional dissection along the common hepatic artery (D1 + β), and extended dissection of nonregional lymph nodes (D2). Eastern Asian surgeons routinely perform extended lymphadenectomy (D2), a practice that some suggest at least partially accounts for the better survival rates in Asian compared with Western series.[35] However, Western studies, including two large, prospective, randomized trials have failed to show a survival benefit with extended lymph node dissection.[36–38] In addition, these trials demonstrated increased postoperative morbidity and mortality associated with more extensive dissections. As a result, an extended lymphadenectomy is typically not performed in most Western countries. In the United States, it is generally accepted to perform an en bloc resection of the regional lymph nodes with the goal of obtaining a minimum of 15 lymph nodes.[25]

OPERATIVE CONSIDERATIONS FOR FORMAL GASTRIC RESECTION
Tumor Location

In general, tumors located in the distal two-thirds of the stomach are best treated with subtotal gastrectomy; whereas, tumors of the proximal one-third of the stomach are treated with total gastrectomy. In Eastern Asia, in an effort to improve the quality of life after gastrectomy, various types of function-preserving laparoscopic gastrectomies have been described for the treatment of EGC. These include proximal gastrectomy, pylorus preserving gastrectomy, and vagus nerve preserved gastrectomy. Laparoscopic proximal gastrectomy has been used to treat ECG tumors located in the proximal third of the stomach.[39] However, this procedure requires an esophagogastrostomy, which is associated with a high rate of gastroesophageal reflux. Laparoscopic pylorus preserving gastrectomy with gastrogastrostomy has been used to treat ECG tumors located in the body of the stomach. This technique has been demonstrated to have satisfactory long-term surgical and oncologic outcomes compared with an open procedure, with potentially lower rates of postgastrectomy dumping syndrome and biliary reflux compared with distal gastrectomy.[40–42] Technical modifications for this procedure include excluding the removal of the prepyloric lymph nodes, assurance of a 4-cm distal margin from the tumor, and a 3- to 4-cm antral cuff for an adequate gastrogastric anastomosis.[30] Given the rarity of ECG in the United States, as well as the limited postoperative data, laparoscopic function-preserving gastrectomies currently have very minimal application in the United States.

Approach

The decision to use a laparoscopic versus an open approach depends on several factors. Principal considerations relate to the technical expertise and experience of the surgeon with advanced minimally invasive techniques. Laparoscopic gastrectomy is a technically challenging operation that requires the skills to perform an adequate lymphadenectomy and an intestinal anastomosis. Relative contraindications for a surgeon who is early in their learning curve include patients with high body mass index (BMI) and advanced tumors, especially those invading surrounding organs requiring en bloc resection. Various technical disadvantages for laparoscopic resection in obese patients have been reported and include decreased surgical visibility, a dissection plane hindered by adipose tissue, and difficulty with anastomoses.[40] Higher BMI has also been reported as an independent risk factor for increased risk of pancreatic fistula following laparoscopic distal gastrectomy.[43] Furthermore, patients with multiple severe comorbidities, those who have received neoadjuvant therapy, or those who have undergone previous laparotomy may not be good candidates for laparoscopic resection early in a surgeon's learning curve.[12] An absolute contraindication is poor cardiopulmonary reserve, due to the decrease in venous return and increase in pulmonary resistance associated with pneumoperitoneum.

Hand-assisted laparoscopic gastrectomy has been advocated by some groups of investigators to overcome the technical challenges associated with a totally laparoscopic approach.[44–47] Laparoscopic gastrectomy is well suited for a hand-assisted approach because an extraction incision is already needed to remove the specimen. Hand-assisted laparoscopic gastrectomy has been shown to maintain the advantages of laparoscopy (less pain, quicker recovery, and shorter hospital stay) while decreasing operative time and minimizing conversions to laparotomy. As with any cancer operation, the safety of the patient and the ability to complete an oncologically sound resection are of paramount concern. Surgeons attempting laparoscopic gastrectomy should have a low threshold for conversion to an open procedure.

Oncologic Concerns

Given the paucity of oncologic outcome data in the United States regarding laparoscopic gastrectomy for gastric cancer, there continues to be significant controversy. As such, caution and meticulous laparoscopic technique must be exercised to adhere to the strict principles of oncologic surgery in patients with potentially curative resections. These principles include minimal tumor manipulation, obtaining negative margins, and performing an adequate lymph node dissection. There also remain questions regarding trocar-site metastasis and the effects of CO_2 pneumoperitoneum. However, there is no good experimental evidence suggesting that CO_2 pneumoperitoneum increases the malignant potential of cancer cells.[48,49] In addition, it has been reported that incisional tumor metastases can occur in 1% of patients with colon cancer following traditional laparotomy,[50] but data exist regarding this risk in gastric cancer. Tumor dissemination and trocar-site metastasis are most likely related to poor technique or advanced disease. Specific technical steps that can be used to prevent trocar site metastasis include (1) minimize handling of the tumor, (2) secure trocars to skin with suture to prevent dislodgement, (3) irrigate the trocar sites with a tumoricidal agent, and (4) use a wound protector at the extraction site. Importantly, the laparoscopic approach must provide oncologic equivalency and must not be a compromise or short-cut procedure.

PATIENT POSITION AND ROOM SETUP

The patient is placed in the supine position with both arms extended (**Fig. 1**). General endotracheal anesthesia is administered. An orogastric tube is placed to decompress the stomach and a Foley catheter is inserted into the bladder. Intravenous antibiotics are administered within 1 hour of the incision. Sequential stockings are applied to the lower extremities for deep venous thrombosis prophylaxis. Additionally, the authors give all patients 5000 units of subcutaneous unfractionated heparin in the preoperative holding area. The patient is secured to the surgical bed to facilitate maximum reverse Trendelenburg position. Additionally, either a bean bag and/or foot board should be used. The video monitors are positioned near the shoulders on each side of the operating table. The surgeon and camera holder stand on the patient's right side. The first-assistant and scrub nurse are positioned on the left side.

The initial trocar is placed approximately 15 cm below the xiphoid in the midline (**Fig. 2**). This can be performed using either a Veress needle or an open Hasson technique, depending on the surgeon's preference and experience. An angled telescope (30° or 45°) should be used to facilitate looking around the corners and to maximize the field of view. Under direct laparoscopic visualization, two additional trocars (5-mm and 12-mm) are placed on each side of the abdomen. A Nathanson liver retractor (Cook Medical, Bloomington, IN, USA) is placed directly through the abdominal wall in the subxiphoid location. The liver retractor is positioned to retract the left lateral segments of the liver to expose the diaphragmatic hiatus. The 12-mm right-sided trocar is the primary operative port and is used to introduce the laparoscopic linear stapler, as well as the EndoStitch (Covidien, Norwalk, CT, USA) or needle holder.

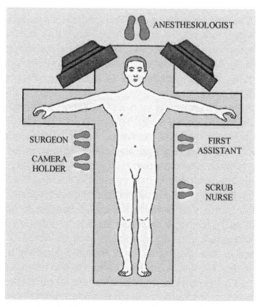

Fig. 1. Operating room setup for laparoscopic gastric resection.

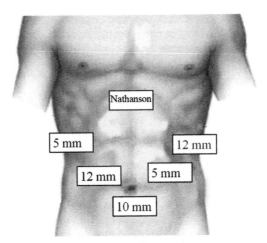

Fig. 2. Trocar placement for laparoscopic gastric resection.

The patient should be positioned in steep reverse Trendelenburg to facilitate exposure of the proximal stomach and the diaphragmatic hiatus.

OPERATIVE TECHNIQUE
Laparoscopic Subtotal Gastrectomy

The first step is to perform a staging laparoscopy (see above) to asses for the potential of curative resection. If the cancer is resectable, the decision is then made as to the feasibility of performing the operation laparoscopically. The laparoscopic procedure begins by retracting the greater omentum cephalad and releasing the omentum from the transverse colon. This is performed with ultrasonic coagulating shears and allows entry into and visualization of the lesser sac. The right gastroepiploic pedicle is followed toward the patient's right side. The pedicle is clipped and ligated close to its origin from the gastroduodenal artery. Attention is then turned to the prepyloric lymph nodes, which are carefully dissected. The proximal duodenum is dissected circumferentially. This is facilitated by the assistant retracting the antrum laterally to linearize the first portion of the duodenum. Careful circumferential retroduodenal dissection just proximal to the duodenal fusion with the head of the pancreas is performed. The duodenum is transected with a reticulating linear 60-mm laparoscopic stapler with a 3.5-mm staple load (**Fig. 3**). This allows for greater mobility and visualization of the right gastric artery and the lymph nodes of the perigastric region and lesser curve. The right gastric artery and associated lymph nodes are divided close to its origin from the hepatic artery proper. If indicated, depending on tumor location, the left gastric vessels are divided near their respective roots with a linear laparoscopic stapler with a vascular cartridge. The proximal site of gastric transection is determined by the location of the tumor. A minimum of 4-cm is needed to assure an adequate proximal margin. As such, for more proximal lesions, it may be necessary to divide the left gastroepiploic artery near its origin, as well as some of the short gastric vessels. The stomach is then transected with multiple (typically 3 or 4) applications of the laparoscopic linear stapler. A 3.5-mm cartridge can often be used in the proximal stomach, whereas a 4.8-mm load may be required for the thicker distal portions. It is important to remove the orogastric tube from the stomach before transection. The specimen is placed in a retrieval bag for later removal.

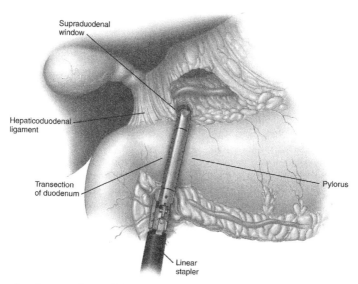

Fig. 3. Duodenal transection with linear stapler. (*From* Parikh M, Pomp A. Laparoscopic total gastrectomy for malignancy. In: Frantzides C, Carlson M, editors. Atlas of minimally invasive surgery. Philadelphia: Saunders, Elsevier, Inc; 2009. p. 43–51; with permission.)

Reconstruction is then accomplished with either a loop (Billroth II) or a Roux-en-Y gastrojejunostomy. This portion of the operation is performed by taking the patient out of reverse Trendelenburg position. A loop gastrojejunostomy is performed by first elevating the transverse mesocolon to identify the ligament of Treitz and selecting a point on the jejunum approximately 30 to 40 cm distally. This point of jejunum is brought over the colon (antecolic) into the lesser sac. If there is undue tension, a window can be made in an avascular area of the transverse mesocolon to allow for a retrocolic passage of the jejunum into the lesser sac. The gastrojejunostomy should be performed on the dependent, posterior wall of the stomach. The anastomosis is performed with a laparoscopic reticulating linear 60-mm stapler. The gastroenterotomy is closed with either interrupted or a running suture.

The Roux-en-Y reconstruction requires identification of the ligament of Treitz and transection of the proximal jejunum 30 to 40 cm distally with a laparoscopic linear stapler. The biliary limb is anastomosed to the jejunum approximately 60 cm distal to the staple line of the Roux limb. The jejunojejunostomy is performed with a laparoscopic linear 60-mm stapler. The enteroenterostomy site is closed transversely with a linear stapler or a hand-sewn technique. Care must be taken to avoid narrowing the Roux limb at this level. The mesenteric defect is closed with suture to prevent internal herniation of the small intestine. The proximal Roux limb is then passed in an antecolic fashion to the lesser sac. If there is undue tension on the Roux limb, it may be passed in a retrocolic position. The gastrojejunostomy should be performed on the dependent, posterior wall of the stomach. The anastomosis is performed with a laparoscopic reticulating linear 60-mm stapler. The gastroenterotomy is closed with either interrupted or a running suture. To test the integrity and patency of the gastrojejunostomy, a flexible upper endoscope is gently advanced across the anastomosis with low insufflation. The gastrojejunostomy is submerged in saline and inspected for air bubbles. A nasogastric tube is positioned in the stomach proximal to the anastomosis. A drain can be placed near the duodenal stump. The specimen is extracted by enlarging the fascia at one of the 12-mm trocar sites. A wound protector (ALEXIS, Applied Medical, Santa Margarita, CA, USA) is used to minimize the risk of tumor implantation at the extraction site. The fascia is closed with a suture passer at all trocar sites larger than 10 mm. Skin incisions are closed with a subcuticular absorbable suture.

Laparoscopic Total Gastrectomy

The procedure for laparoscopic total gastrectomy for cancer begins with a staging laparoscopy and is similar to that described above for subtotal gastrectomy. However, a total gastrectomy requires complete mobilization of the gastric fundus and complete dissection of the diaphragmatic hiatus with circumferential dissection of the distal esophagus into the mediastinum. The mobilization of the gastric fundus is performed by dividing all of the short gastric vessels with ultrasonic coagulating shears. The dissection continues medially around the tip of the fundus to fully visualize the left crus of the diaphragm. This is facilitated by retracting the fundus inferiorly and toward the patient's right side to expose and divide any posterior gastric attachments. The gastrohepatic omentum is completely divided with ultrasonic coagulating shears to the level of the right crus. The dissection is continued anteriorly by dividing the phrenoesophageal ligament with ultrasonic shears. A plane is then developed between the right crus and the esophagus. The surgeon's left-hand instrument retracts the crus laterally and the right-hand instrument gently sweeps the esophagus and periesophageal tissue to the left to bluntly mobilize the distal esophagus. This dissection is carried high into the mediastinum. Posterior segmental arteries from the aorta are divided with ultrasonic shears. The tissue attached to the medial border of the base of the right crus is divided until the origin of the right crus from the left crus is visualized from the right side of the esophagus. Similarly, on the left side, the left crus is bluntly dissected from the esophagus. The dissection is again carried into the mediastinum and connected with the dissection from the right. The medial border of the left crus is dissected back to its junction with the right crus, joining the plane previously begun from the right side. A large window is thereby created posterior to the esophagus and proximal stomach and anterior to both crura. A Penrose drain is then looped around the gastroesophageal junction to provide retraction and improved exposure. It is important that the hiatal dissection is a dissection of the crura and not, per se, a dissection of the esophagus. Once the esophagus is fully mobilized it is divided with a laparoscopic reticulating linear stapler.

Reconstruction is accomplished with a Roux-en-Y esophagojejunostomy. Creation of the Roux limb occurs as described above. The esophagojejunal anastomosis can then be created with a circular stapler, linear stapler, or hand-sewn technique. The authors prefer to use a circular stapler, which involves a prepackaged flipped, 25-mm anvil secured to the distal end of an orogastric tube (OrVil, Covidien, Norwalk, CT, USA). The proximal end of the orogastric tube is carefully passed transorally down the esophagus to the level of the esophageal staple line. A small enterotomy is made near the esophageal staple line and the proximal end of the orogastric tube is grasped and pulled through the enterotomy while the anvil is simultaneously guided through the oropharynx and hypopharynx. Passage of the anvil through the hypopharynx requires great care to prevent perforation. To facilitate safe passage of the anvil, the patient's neck should be extended and an anterior jaw-lift maneuver performed. Resistance of the anvil is usually encountered at the level of the cricopharyngeus muscle, the narrowest point of passage. However, constant gentle pressure of the anvil against the cricopharyngeus muscle will promote relaxation of the muscle and allow safe passage into the esophagus. The orogastric tube is pulled until the stem of the anvil emerges from the esophagotomy. The suture along the stem of the anvil is then cut to allow the anvil to flip back into standard position. The orogastric tube is released from the stem of the anvil and removed. An enterotomy is created at the staple line of the Roux limb. The 12-mm trocar in the left lateral upper abdomen is removed and the circular stapler is passed into the peritoneal cavity directly through the abdominal wall. The circular stapler is inserted into the enterotomy of the Roux limb and advanced approximately 5 to 10 cm. The spike of the stapler is advanced through the antimesenteric border of the jejunum and united with the stem of the anvil (**Fig. 4**). The stapler is closed into range and then fired to create a 25-mm (16.9 mm inner diameter) circular esophagojejunostomy. The stapler is carefully removed and both doughnuts are inspected. The overhang portion of the Roux limb is resected with a linear stapler, thereby eliminating the previously made enterotomy. The esophagojejunostomy is reinforced with two seromuscular sutures at the 3 and 9 o'clock positions. The proximal Roux limb is cross-clamped with an atraumatic bowel clamp and a final endoscopy is performed to rule out a leak. Specimen extraction and wound closure are performed as previously described.

OUTCOMES

Numerous retrospective analyses have shown that laparoscopic gastric resection for malignancy is both feasible and safe, with no increased morbidity when compared with open resection. Several prospective, randomized studies are confirmatory (**Table 1**).[4,51–56] A prospective, multicenter, randomized clinical trial is underway to

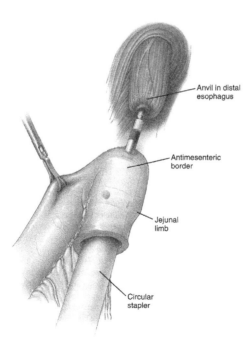

Anvil in distal
esophagus

Antimesenteric
border

Jejunal
limb

Circular
stapler

Fig. 4. Creation of esophagojejunostomy with a 25-mm circular stapler. (*From* Parikh M, Pomp A. Laparoscopic total gastrectomy for malignancy. In: Frantzides C, Carlson M, editors. Atlas of minimally invasive surgery. Philadelphia: Saunders, Elsevier, Inc; 2009. p. 43–51; with permission.)

Table 1
Prospective, randomized studies evaluating laparoscopic-assisted and open gastric resection for gastric cancer

Author	Year	Procedure	Patients (n) Lap	Open	Findings in Laparoscopic Group
Kitano et al[51]	2002	LADG vs ODG	14	14	Improved EBL, ambulation, ROBF
Hyashi et al[52]	2005	LADG vs ODG	14	14	Improved epidural use, ROBF; shorter LOS
Lee and Han[53]	2005	LADG vs ODG	24	23	Longer OR time; trend toward less pain medication and LOS
Huscher et al[4]	2005	LSG vs OSG	30	29	Improved EBL; similar morbidity, mortality, 5-y OS and DFS
Kim et al[54]	2008	LADG vs ODG	82	82	Less EBL and pain medication; shorter LOS
Kim et al[55]	2010	LADG vs ODG	179	161	Similar morbidity and mortality
Cai et al[56]	2011	LAG vs OG	61	62	Similar morbidity and OS at 2 y

Abbreviations: DFS, disease-free survival; EBL, estimated blood loss; LADG, laparoscopy-assisted distal gastrectomy; LAG, laparoscopy-assisted gastrectomy; LOS, length of stay; LSG, laparoscopic subtotal; ODG, open distal gastrectomy; OG, open gastrectomy; OR, operating room; OS, overall survival; OSG, open subtotal gastrectomy; ROBF, return of bowel function.

assess the short-term and long-term outcomes of laparoscopic gastrectomy for EGC. Although final results from the Korean Laparoscopic Gastro-intestinal Surgery Study (KLASS) Group trial have not yet been published, interim results demonstrate no difference in postoperative complication rates (10.5% vs 14.7%, $P = .14$) or mortality (1.1% vs 0%, $P = .50$) between the laparoscopic and open groups, respectively.[55] In the only prospective, randomized trial published from the West, Huscher and colleagues[4] demonstrated decreased intraoperative blood loss, earlier PO intake, and reduced length of hospital stay in patients randomized to laparoscopic-assisted subtotal gastrectomy compared with an open procedure. Furthermore, there was no difference in the mean number of lymph nodes harvested between the open and laparoscopic groups (33 ± 17 vs 30 ± 15, respectively), indicating adequate staging. Ikeda and colleagues[57] recently reported less blood loss and shorter length of stay with no difference in complication rates for patients treated with a totally laparoscopic distal gastrectomy compared with a laparoscopic-assisted procedure. Similarly, investigators from the United States have demonstrated less blood loss, earlier return of bowel function, equivalent lymph node harvest, and shorter postoperative length of stay.[58–62] Also, Western data are becoming more robust (**Table 2**).[63–68] However, these benefits come at the cost of significantly longer operating times for laparoscopic resections, especially early in a surgeon's learning curve. For laparoscopic distal gastrectomy, the most commonly performed laparoscopic procedure, conversion rates reported in the literature range from 2.3% to 25%, with the most common reason for conversion being extent of disease, not intraoperative complications.[69]

Common intraoperative complications that can occur with these procedures include retraction injuries to adjacent tissues or organs (such as the pancreas, spleen, liver, and esophagus) and bleeding (commonly from the right gastroepiploic vessels during infrapyloric dissection, or the common hepatic or splenic vessels during lymphadenectomy).[12] Perioperative complication rates (within 30 days) for laparoscopic distal gastrectomy reported in the literature commonly range between 10% and 20% in

Table 2
Western studies comparing laparoscopic and open gastric resection for gastric carcinoma perioperative outcomes

Author	Year	Country	Total Patients	Laparoscopic Group (n)	Open Group (n)	Laparoscopic Procedure	Laparoscopic Lymph Node Harvest (n)[a]	Laparoscopic Op Time (min)[a]	Laparoscopic EBL (mL)[a]	Laparoscopic LOS (days)[a]	Laparoscopic 30-d Morbidity	Laparoscopic 30-d Morbidity (%)
Reyes et al[58]	2001	USA	36	18	18	Distal	8 (4–14)	252 (120–366)	209 (30–400)	6.3 ± NR	NR	0.0%
Weber et al[61]	2003	USA	25	12	13	Distal	8 (4–14)	252 (132–366)	230 (30–400)	6.3 ± NR	NR	0.0%
Huscher et al[4]	2005	Italy	59	30	29	Subtotal	30 ± 15	196 ± 21	229 ± 144	10.3 ± 3.6	26.7%	3.3%
Dulucq et al[63]	2005	France	52	24	28	Total (8) and partial (16)	24 ± 12 & 17 ± 7	183 ± 48 & 130 ± 31	81 ± 107 & 60 ± 90	16.9 ± 3 & 16 ± 5.4	0% & 12.5%	0.0%
Varela et al[62]	2006	USA	36	15	21	Various	15 ± 9	244 ± 95	138 ± 114	NR	7.0%	0.0%
Pugliese et al[64]	2007	Italy	147	48	99	Total (4) and subtotal (43)	32 ± 9	240 ± 23	150 ± 85	10 ± 3	10.0%	2.0%
Strong et al[59]	2009	USA	60	30	30	Subtotal	18 (7–36)	270[b] (150–485)	200[b] (50–800)	5[b] (2–26)	26.0%	0.0%
Guzman et al[60]	2009	USA	78	30	48	Total (4) and partial (26)	24 ± 8	399 ± 85	200 (50–900)	7[b] (3–32)	30.0%	0.0%
Sica et al[65]	2011	Italy	47	22	25	Total (5) and subtotal (17)	29 ± 7	NR	NR	NR	NR	NR
Moisan et al[66]	2011	Chile	62	31	31	Total (22) and subtotal (9)	35[b] (23–53)	250[b] (160–420)	100[b] (50–500)	7[b] (4–59)	22.5%	0.0%
Scatizzi et al[67]	2011	Italy	60	30	30	Subtotal	31[b] (16–60)	240 ± 65	NR	7[b] (6–50)	13.3%	0.0%
Orsenigo et al[68]	2011	Italy	378	109	269	Total (17) and distal (92)	31 ± 14	272 ± 74	170 ± 199	13 ± 9	26.0%	0.0%

Abbreviation: NR, not reported.
[a] mean ± SD or (range) unless otherwise noted.
[b] Median (range).

Eastern countries, and between 20% and 30% in Western countries.[12] It is possible that these differences relate to the older, heavier population seen in Western countries that often have increased comorbidities. Potential complications include anastomotic leak (1%–2% for subtotal and 5–15% for total gastrectomy), hemorrhage (approximately 1%), delayed gastric emptying (approximately 1%), and wound complications (approximately 2%).[12,70,71] A recent meta-analysis of laparoscopic versus open distal gastrectomy for early-stage cancer concluded that the laparoscopic approach demonstrated decreased blood loss intraoperatively, earlier postoperative flatus, and shorter hospital stay, but a smaller number of lymph nodes harvested and longer operating times than open operations.[72] A separate meta-analysis concluded that laparoscopic surgery for advanced gastric cancer resulted in longer operating times, less blood loss, shorter hospital stay, and comparable number of dissected lymph nodes.[73] A third meta-analysis that included patients regardless of stage concluded that laparoscopic distal gastrectomy was associated with lower overall complications, estimated blood loss, and hospital stay; clinically comparable lymph node harvest; but longer operative times.[74] In this analysis, there was no significant difference in mortality or major complications between the two groups.

Several studies have recently been published evaluating long-term survival. Lee and colleagues[30] reported a 5-year survival rate of 93.4% in 511 patients with early gastric cancer treated laparoscopically, which is comparable with open resection. Pak and colleagues[75] reported 5-year survival of 96% for stage I and 83% for stage II patients treated with laparoscopic resection. Other studies have similarly shown equivalent oncologic outcomes between laparoscopic and open gastric resections for early gastric cancer.[4,76] Evidence for the long-term comparability of laparoscopic resection for advanced gastric cancer is now beginning to emerge.[4,32,33,65] In a retrospective study of 239 patients with a median follow-up of 55 months, overall 5-year survival was 78.8% and disease-specific survival was 85.6%.[32] In this study, survival was highly correlated with TNM stage, with IB having a 90.5% survival dropping to 36.5% for stage IIIC.

THE LEARNING CURVE

The technical skill needed to complete complex laparoscopic resections is a sine qua non. Factors affecting one's ability to master these advanced operations include dexterity, training, personal experience, patient volume, and extent of disease treated, as well as hospital factors such as available equipment and familiarity of the surgical team. An analysis by Zhang and Tanigawa[77] revealed that 60 to 90 cases of laparoscopic gastrectomy are required to complete learning. These numbers, however, may be an underestimate in patients with more advanced stages of disease that require a more technically demanding, expanded lymphadenectomy. A study by Jin and colleagues[78] found that after achieving competency with laparoscopic distal gastrectomy for EGC, additional experience was required to master the added complexity of an extensive lymph node dissection for more advanced cancers. Furthermore, a review of hospital volume and operating room time revealed that longer operative time was associated with an increased risk of complications.[79] In this study, hospitals defined as having a high volume of laparoscopic gastrectomies had a modest positive effect on operating room time, highlighting the importance of a cohesive surgical team that is familiar with performing these procedures.

EMERGING TECHNOLOGY

There are emerging minimally invasive techniques that may offer solutions to the technical limitations of conventional laparoscopic surgery. Robotic surgery for gastric cancer has the potential benefits of three-dimensional imaging, elimination of resting tremor, ergonomic comfort, and greater control in fine manipulation when performing extensive lymph node dissections or intracorporeal anastomoses. However, the lack of tactile sense and limitations in macroscopic manipulation speeds and shift of scene may offer experienced surgeons who have mastered laparoscopy no real advantage.[80] Reports of the feasibility of robotic surgery for gastric cancer are beginning to emerge.[81–83] However, the long-term results of this technique and whether sufficient benefits to patients exist to justify the additional costs have yet to be confirmed. Finally, a report of single-incision laparoscopic distal gastrectomy for early gastric cancer in seven subjects has recently been published.[84] The investigators concluded that the technique was safe and feasible and allowed for a sufficient lymph node harvest, but further evaluation of this technique is needed.

SUMMARY

Gastric cancer remains a common disease worldwide. Diversity of tumor location and disease stage remain polarized between Asian and Western countries. Furthermore, Western patients are more likely to have a higher BMI and increased numbers of comorbidities that may make laparoscopic resections more challenging. Multiple prospective, randomized trials from Asia have demonstrated the benefits (faster recovery and shorter hospital stay) of laparoscopic gastrectomy for EGC while maintaining equivalent short-term and long-term oncologic outcomes compared with open surgery. Data regarding the long-term outcomes of laparoscopy in advanced disease are becoming more robust and seem to offer equivalent results to open surgery. In the United States, laparoscopic gastrectomy for cancer remains in its infancy and somewhat controversial. To date, reports of laparoscopic gastrectomy for cancer from the United States suffer from uncontrolled design, small numbers, or limited follow-up. However, various groups continue to investigate and advance laparoscopic gastrectomy for gastric cancer. In addition, several randomized, controlled trials are ongoing, which will further help define patient selection and outcomes. It seems that laparoscopic gastrectomy will continue to evolve in the United States. It is likely that new technologies will be developed that shorten the extensive learning curve required to master these complex minimally invasive procedures.

REFERENCES

1. Kitano S, Iso Y, Moriyama M, et al. Laparoscopy-assisted Billroth I gastrectomy. Surg Laparosc Endosc 1994;4(2):146–8.
2. Azagra JS, Goergen M, De Simone P, et al. Minimally invasive surgery for gastric cancer. Surg Endosc 1999;13(4):351–7.
3. Azagra JS, Goergen M, Gilbart E, et al. Laparoscopy-assisted total gastrectomy with extended lymphadenectomy for cancer: technical aspects. Le Jour Coeliochir 2001;40:35–6.
4. Huscher CG, Mingoli A, Sgarzini G, et al. Laparoscopic versus open subtotal gastrectomy for distal gastric cancer: five-year results of a randomized prospective trial. Ann Surg 2005;241(2):232–7.
5. Weeks JC, Nelson H, Gelber S, et al. Short-term quality-of-life outcomes following laparoscopic-assisted colectomy vs open colectomy for colon cancer: a randomized trial. JAMA 2002;287(3):321–8.
6. Buunen M, Veldkamp R, Hop WC, et al. Survival after laparoscopic surgery versus open surgery for colon cancer: long-term outcome of a randomised clinical trial. Lancet Oncol 2009;10(1):44–52.

7. Angst E, Hiatt JR, Gloor B, et al. Laparoscopic surgery for cancer: a systematic review and a way forward. J Am Coll Surg 2010;211(3):412–23.

8. Gotoda T, Yanagisawa A, Sasako M, et al. Incidence of lymph node metastasis from early gastric cancer: estimation with a large number of cases at two large centers. Gastric Cancer 2000;3(4):219–25.

9. Jemal A, Bray F, Center MM, et al. Global cancer statistics. CA Cancer J Clin 2011;61(2):69–90.

10. American Cancer Society. What Are the Key Statistics About Stomach Cancer? 2011. Available at: http://www.cancer.org/Cancer/StomachCancer/DetailedGuide/stomach-cancer-key-statistics. Accessed September 29, 2012.

11. Al-Refaie WB, Abdalla EK, Ahmed SA, et al. Gastric cancer. In: Feig BW, Berger DH, Fuhrman GH, editors. The MD Anderson surgical Oncology Handbook. 4th edition. Philadelphia: Lippincott William & Wilkins; 2006. p. 205–40.

12. Strong VE. Laparoscopic resection for gastric carcinoma: Western experience. Surg Onc Clin N Am 2012;21(1):141–58.

13. Siewert JR. Gastric cancer: the dispute between East and West. Gastric Cancer 2005;8(2):59–61.

14. Griffin SM. Gastric cancer in the East: same disease, different patient. Br J Surg 2005;92(9):1055–6.

15. Edge SB, Byrd DR, Compton CC, et al, editors. American Joint Committee on Cancer Staging Manual. 7th edition. New York: Springer.

16. Japanese Gastric Cancer Association. Japanese classification of gastric carcinoma: 3rd English edition. Gastric Cancer 2011;14(2):101–12.

17. Goldfarb M, Brower S, Schwaitzberg SD. Minimally invasive surgery and cancer: controversies part 1. Surg Endosc 2010;24(2):304–34.

18. Bentrem D, Gerdes H, Tang L, et al. Clinical correlation of endoscopic ultrasonography with pathologic stage and outcome in patients undergoing curative resection for gastric cancer. Ann Surg Oncol 2007;14(6):1853–9.

19. Ott K, Lordick F, Blank S, et al. Gastric cancer: surgery in 2011. Langenbecks Arch Surg 2011;396(6):743–58.

20. Power DG, Schattner MA, Gerdes H, et al. Endoscopic ultrasound can improve the selection for laparoscopy in patients with localized gastric cancer. J Am Coll Surg 2009;208(2):173–8.

21. Samee A, Moorthy K, Jaipersad T, et al. Evaluation of the role of laparoscopic ultrasonography in the staging of oesophagogastric cancers. Surg Endosc 2009;23(9):2061–5.

22. Shimizu H, Imamura H, Ohta K, et al. Usefulness of staging laparoscopy for advanced gastric cancer. Surg Today 2010;40(2):119–24.

23. Bentrem D, Wilton A, Mazumdar M, et al. The value of peritoneal cytology as a preoperative predictor in patients with gastric carcinoma undergoing a curative resection. Ann Surg Oncol 2005;12(5):347–53.

24. Mezhir JJ, Shah MA, Jacks LM, et al. Positive peritoneal cytology in patients with gastric cancer: natural history and outcome of 291 patients. Ann Surg Oncol 2010;17(12):3173–80.

25. National Comprehensive Cancer Network (NCCN) clinical practice guidelines in oncology: gastric cancer (V.2.2011). National Comprehensive Cancer Network; 2010. Available at: NCCN.org. Accessed September 29, 2012.

26. Nozaki I, Kubo Y, Kurita A, et al. Long-term outcome after laparoscopic wedge resection for early gastric cancer. Surg Endosc 2008;22(12):2665–9.

27. Kobayashi T, Kazui T, Kimura T. Surgical local resection for early gastric cancer. Surg Laparosc Endosc Percutan Tech 2003;13(5):299–303.

28. Ludwig K, Klautke G, Bernhard J, et al. Minimally invasive and local treatment for mucosal early gastric cancer. Surg Endosc 2005;19(10):1362–6.
29. Tanimura S, Higashino M, Fukunaga Y, et al. Laparoscopic gastrectomy for gastric cancer: experience with more than 600 cases. Surg Endosc 2008;22(5):1161–4.
30. Lee SW, Nomura E, Bouras G, et al. Long-term oncologic outcomes from laparoscopic gastrectomy for gastric cancer: a single-center experience of 601 consecutive resections. J Am Coll Surg 2010;211(1):33–40.
31. Huscher GC, Mingoli A, Sgarzini G, et al. Extended indications of laparoscopic procedures to advanced gastric cancer. Surg Endosc 2005;19(5):737.
32. Park DJ, Han SU, Hyung WJ, et al. Long-term outcomes after laparoscopy-assisted gastrectomy for advanced gastric cancer: a large-scale multicenter retrospective study. Surg Endosc 2012;26(6):1548–53.
33. Hamabe A, Omori T, Tanaka K, et al. Comparison of long-term results between laparoscopy-assisted gastrectomy and open gastrectomy with D2 lymph node dissection for advanced gastric cancer. Surg Endosc 2012;26(6):1702–9.
34. Huang JL, Wei HB, Zheng ZH, et al. Laparoscopy-assisted D2 radical distal gastrectomy for advanced gastric cancer. Dig Surg 2010;27(4):291–6.
35. de Bree E, Charalampakis V, Melissas J, et al. The extent of lymph node dissection for gastric cancer: a critical appraisal. J Surg Oncol 2010;102(6):552–62.
36. Dent DM, Madden MV, Price SK. Randomized comparison of R1 and R2 gastrectomy for gastric carcinoma. Br J Surg 1988;75(2):110–2.
37. Cuschieri A, Weeden S, Fielding J, et al. Patient survival after D1 and D2 resections for gastric cancer: long-term results of the MRC randomized surgical trial. Surgical Co-operative Group. Br J Cancer 1999;79(9–10):1522–30.
38. Hartgrink HH, van de Velde CJ, Putter H, et al. Extended lymph node dissection for gastric cancer: who may benefit? Final results of the randomized Dutch gastric cancer group trial. J Clin Oncol 2004;22(11):2069–77.
39. Tanimura S, Higashino M, Fukunaga Y, et al. Laparoscopic gastrectomy with regional lymph node dissection for upper gastric cancer. Br J Surg 2007;94(2):204–7.
40. Koeda K, Nishizuka S, Wakabayashi G. Minimally invasive surgery for gastric cancer: the future standard of care. World J Surg 2011;35(7):1469–77.
41. Jiang X, Hiki N, Nunobe S, et al. Long-term outcome and survival with laparoscopy-assisted pylorus-preserving gastrectomy for early gastric cancer. Surg Endosc 2011;25(4):1182–6.
42. Horiuchi T, Shimomatsuya T, Chiba Y. Laparoscopically assisted pylorus-preserving gastrectomy. Surg Endosc 2001;15(3):325–8.
43. Jiang X, Hiki N, Nunobe S, et al. Postoperative pancreatic fistula and the risk factors of laparoscopy-assisted distal gastrectomy for early gastric cancer. Ann Surg Oncol 2012;19(1):115–21.
44. Sakuramoto S, Kikuchi S, Kuroyama S, et al. Laparoscopy-assisted distal gastrectomy for early gastric cancer: experience with 111 consecutive patients. Surg Endosc 2006;20(1):55–60.
45. Tanimura S, Higashino M, Fukunaga Y, et al. Hand-assisted laparoscopic distal gastrectomy with regional lymph node dissection for gastric cancer. Surg Laparosc Endosc Percutan Tech 2001;11(3):155–60.
46. Chau CH, Siu WT, Li MK. Hand-assisted D2 subtotal gastrectomy for carcinoma of stomach. Surg Laparosc Endosc Percutan Tech 2002;12(4):268–72.
47. Kim YW, Bae JM, Lee JH, et al. The role of hand-assisted laparoscopic distal gastrectomy for distal gastric cancer. Surg Endosc 2005;19(1):29–33.
48. Are C, Talamini MA. Laparoscopy and malignancy. J Laparoendosc Adv Surg Tech A 2005;15(1):38–47.

49. Jingli C, Rong C, Rubai X. Influence of colorectal laparoscopic surgery on dissemination and seeding of tumor cells. Surg Endosc 2006;20(11):1759–61.
50. Reilly WT, Nelson H, Schroeder G, et al. Wound recurrence following conventional treatment of colorectal cancer. A rare but perhaps underestimated problem. Dis Colon Rectum 1996;39(2):200–7.
51. Kitano S, Shiraishi N, Fujii K, et al. A randomized controlled trial comparing open vs laparoscopy-assisted distal gastrectomy for the treatment of early gastric cancer: an interim report. Surgery 2002;131(Suppl 1):S306–11.
52. Hayashi H, Ochiai T, Shimada H, et al. Prospective randomized study of open versus laparoscopy-assisted distal gastrectomy with extraperigastric lymph node dissection for early gastric cancer. Surg Endosc 2005;19(9): 1172–6.
53. Lee JH, Han HS. A prospective randomized study comparing open vs laparoscopy-assisted distal gastrectomy in early gastric cancer: early results. Surg Endosc 2005;19(2):168–73.
54. Kim YW, Baik YH, Yun YH, et al. Improved quality of life outcomes after laparoscopy-assisted distal gastrectomy for early gastric cancer: results of a prospective randomized clinical trial. Ann Surg 2008;248(5):721–7.
55. Kim HH, Hyung WJ, Cho GS, et al. Morbidity and mortality of laparoscopic gastrectomy versus open gastrectomy for gastric cancer: an interim report—a phase III multicenter, prospective, randomized trial (KLASS Trial). Ann Surg 2010;251(3):417–20.
56. Cai J, Wei D, Gao CF, et al. A prospective randomized study comparing open versus laparoscopy-assisted D2 radical gastrectomy in advanced gastric cancer. Dig Surg 2011;28(5–6):331–7.
57. Ikeda O, Sakaguchi Y, Aoki Y, et al. Advantages of totally laparoscopic distal gastrectomy over laparoscopically assisted distal gastrectomy for gastric cancer. Surg Endosc 2009;23(10):2374–9.
58. Reyes CD, Weber KJ, Gagner M, et al. Laparoscopic vs open gastrectomy. A retrospective review. Surg Endosc 2001;15(9):928–31.
59. Strong VE, Devaud N, Allen PJ, et al. Laparoscopic versus open subtotal gastrectomy for adenocarcinoma: a case-control study. Ann Surg Oncol 2009;16(6): 1507–13.
60. Guzman EA, Pigazzi A, Lee B, et al. Totally laparoscopic gastric resection with extended lymphadenectomy for gastric adenocarcinoma. Ann Surg Oncol 2009;16(8):2218–23.
61. Weber KJ, Reyes CD, Gagner M, et al. Comparison of laparoscopic and open gastrectomy for malignant disease. Surg Endosc 2003;17(6):968–71.
62. Varela JE, Hiyashi M, Nguyen T, et al. Comparison of laparoscopic and open gastrectomy for gastric cancer. Am J Surg 2006;192(6):837–42.
63. Dulucq JL, Wintringer P, Stabilini C, et al. Laparoscopic and open gastric resections for malignant lesions: a prospective comparative study. Surg Endosc 2005; 19(7):933–8.
64. Pugliese R, Maggioni D, Sansonna F, et al. Total and subtotal laparoscopic gastrectomy for adenocarcinoma. Surg Endosc 2007;21(1):21–7.
65. Sica GS, Iaculli E, Biancone L, et al. Comparative study of laparoscopic vs open gastrectomy in gastric cancer management. World J Gastroenterol 2011;17(41): 4602–6.
66. Moisan F, Norero E, Slako M, et al. Completely laparoscopic versus open gastrectomy for early and advanced gastric cancer: a matched cohort study. Surg Endosc 2012;26(3):661–72.

67. Scatizzi M, Kroning KC, Lenzi E, et al. Laparoscopic versus open distal gastrectomy for locally advanced gastric cancer: a case-control study. Updates Surg 2011;63(1):17–23.
68. Orsenigo E, Di Palo S, Tamburini A, et al. Laparoscopy-assisted gastrectomy versus open gastrectomy for gastric cancer: a monoinstitutional Western center experience. Surg Endosc 2011;25(1):140–5.
69. Shiraishi N, Yasuda K, Kitano S. Laparoscopic gastrectomy with lymph node dissection for gastric cancer. Gastric Cancer 2006;9(3):167–76.
70. Bo T, Zhihong P, Peiwu Y, et al. General complications following laparoscopic-assisted gastrectomy and analysis of techniques to manage them. Surg Endosc 2009;23(8):1860–5.
71. Kitano S, Shiraishi N. Current status of laparoscopic gastrectomy for cancer in Japan. Surg Endosc 2004;18(2):182–5.
72. Peng JS, Song H, Yang ZL, et al. Meta-analysis of laparoscopy-assisted distal gastrectomy and conventional open distal gastrectomy for early gastric cancer. Chin J Cancer 2010;29(4):349–54.
73. Martinez-Ramos D, Miralles-Tena JM, Cuesta MA, et al. Laparoscopy versus open surgery for advanced and resectable gastric cancer: a meta-analysis. Rev Esp Enferm Dig 2011;103(3):133–41.
74. Vinuela EF, Gonen M, Brennan MF, et al. Laparoscopic versus open distal gastrectomy for gastric cancer: a meta-analysis of randomized controlled trials and high-quality nonrandomized studies. Ann Surg 2012;255(3):446–56.
75. Pak KH, Hyung WJ, Son T, et al. Long-term oncologic outcomes of 714 consecutive laparoscopic gastrectomies for gastric cancer: results from the 7-year experience of a single institute. Surg Endosc 2012;26(1):130–6.
76. Song J, Lee HJ, Cho GS, et al. Recurrence following laparoscopy-assisted gastrectomy for gastric cancer: a multicenter retrospective analysis of 1,417 patients. Ann Surg Oncol 2010;17(7):1777–86.
77. Zhang X, Tanigawa N. Learning curve of laparoscopic surgery for gastric cancer, a laparoscopic distal gastrectomy-based analysis. Surg Endosc 2009;23(6): 1259–64.
78. Jin SH, Kim DY, Kim H, et al. Multidimensional learning curve in laparoscopy-assisted gastrectomy for early gastric cancer. Surg Endosc 2007;21(1):28–33.
79. Kuwabara K, Matsuda S, Fushimi K, et al. Hospital volume and quality of laparoscopic gastrectomy in Japan. Dig Surg 2009;26(5):422–9.
80. Kim HH, Ahn SH. The current status and future perspectives of laparoscopic surgery for gastric cancer. J Korean Surg Soc 2011;81(3):151–62.
81. Song J, Oh SJ, Kang WH, et al. Robot-assisted gastrectomy with lymph node dissection for gastric cancer: lessons learned from an initial 100 consecutive procedures. Ann Surg 2009;249(6):927–32.
82. Eom BW, Yoon HM, Ryu KW, et al. Comparison of surgical performance and short-term clinical outcomes between laparoscopic and robotic surgery in distal gastric cancer. Eur J Surg Oncol 2012;38(1):57–63.
83. Lee HH, Hur H, Jung H, et al. Robot-assisted distal gastrectomy for gastric cancer: initial experience. Am J Surg 2011;201(6):841–5.
84. Omori T, Oyama T, Akamatsu H, et al. Transumbilical single-incision laparoscopic distal gastrectomy for early gastric cancer. Surg Endosc 2011;25(7):2400–4.

Laparoscopic Distal Pancreatectomy

Omar Yusef Kudsi, MD, MBA[a],*, Michel Gagner, MD[b],
Daniel B. Jones, MD, MS[a]

KEYWORDS

- Laparoscopic approach • Pancreatectomy • Pancreatic fistula
- Pancreatic adenocarcinoma

KEY POINTS

- Laparoscopic distal pancreatectomy (LDP) is a safe procedure with a morbidity rate comparable to that of open distal pancreatectomy (ODP).
- Pancreatic surgeons should report their outcome diligently (resection margin, lymph node count, and morbidity rate, including pancreatic fistula), and survival with the importance of following International Study Group on Pancreatic Fistula (ISGPF) guidelines.
- Selective ligation of the main pancreatic duct remains a challenging step in the laparoscopic approach and it may decrease fistula rate.
- The role and oncologic safety of LDP for pancreatic adenocarcinoma or mucinous cystadenocarcinoma remain unknown.
- LDP with spleen preservation can be considered a matter of surgical preference and is not recommended in cases of suspected or confirmed adenocarcinoma of the body/tail of the pancreas or in cases of splenic vessels encasement.

INTRODUCTION

Laparoscopic approach for benign and malignant lesions in the tail of the pancreas is becoming a more widely used approach. Multiple prospective studies have shown the feasibility and safety of LDP in single-center and multicenter settings.[1–3] Distal pancreatectomy (DP) is defined as the resection of the body/tail of the pancreas to the left of the superior mesenteric vein. LDP is a challenging procedure, because the pancreas is surrounded by critical structures and located in the retroperitoneum. Mishandling the pancreas itself can be unforgiving and may result in iatrogenic injury that may increase the risk of complications, such as pancreatic fistula. Distal pancreatic adenocarcinoma is an aggressive tumor and may not be appropriate for the laparoscopic

[a] Department of Surgery, Beth Israel Deaconess Medical Center, Harvard Medical School, 330 Brookline Avenue, Boston, MA 02215, USA; [b] Minimally Invasive Surgery Section, Clinique Michel Gagner, Inc., 315 Place D'Youville, Montreal, QC H2Y 0A4, Canada
* Corresponding author.
E-mail address: okudsi@bidmc.harvard.edu

Surg Oncol Clin N Am 22 (2013) 59–73
http://dx.doi.org/10.1016/j.soc.2012.08.003
1055-3207/13/$ – see front matter © 2013 Elsevier Inc. All rights reserved.

surgonc.theclinics.com

approach, especially because many pancreatic surgeons are not taught to perform advanced laparoscopy during their residency training.

DIAGNOSIS AND STAGING

Early reports of laparoscopic pancreas resections focused on staging. The use of pancreatic protocol CT scan, has limited the need for staging laparoscopy. Staging laparoscopy using intraoperative ultrasonography may assess vascular tumor involvement and local respectability but no comparative data exist to describe the advantages of this approach over staging CT scan.

A tissue diagnosis is required in specific cases where preoperative or palliative chemotherapy is considered part of the treatment of pancreatic cancer. Endoscopic ultrasonography fine-needle aspiration (EUS-FNA), cystic fluid sampling, and endoscopic retrograde cholangiopancreatography (ERCP) are the most common options for pancreatic tissue biopsy. ERCP may be useful for evaluating the ductal anatomy and its relation to the lesion. Alternatively, magnetic resonance cholangiopancreatography is a noninvasive study to evaluate the pancreatic anatomy. EUS-FNA is the most reliable and accurate method of obtaining tissue. Lennon and colleagues[4] described their EUS-guided tattooing technique before LDP. EUS-guided tattooing was feasible in all 13 cases (EUS-guided tattooing to surgery, mean 20.3 days). The tattoo was visible in all cases with no significant complications associated with this technique. Newman and colleagues[5] reviewed the safety and efficacy of preoperative EUS-guided tattooing. Ten patients underwent preoperative EUS-guided tattoo and the lesions were identified intraoperatively. The nontattoo group (26 patients) had variable success and 1 patient required a repeat operative procedure because of inability to identify 8-mm insulinoma. More studies are needed to identify the role of EUS-guided tattooing. The potential of decreasing operative time and demarcating a precise line of resection for laparoscopic surgeons makes this procedure attractive for small pancreatic lesions.

SELECTION CRITERIA

LDP for appropriate distal pancreatic neoplasms includes all benign lesions and neoplasms without metastasis or local invasion (ie, colon or stomach invasion or encasement of adjacent major vessels, such as common hepatic artery, superior mesenteric artery, celiac axis, and portal vein).

In general, patients should be less than 80 years of age and have been diagnosed with lesions in the pancreatic body/tail localized pancreatic cancer ($\leq$T3) without evidence of distant metastasis, peritoneal seeding, or para-aortic lymph node metastasis. Cases with high malignant potential, such as invasive ductal cancer and mucinous cystic neoplasm, should be treated with en bloc resection of the spleen. Islet cell tumor and cystic diseases other than mucinous cystic neoplasm can be treated with spleen-sparing LDP. Patients needing venous resection were considered candidates for resection. In addition, surgery may be appropriate when R0 resection is expected from combined resection of adjacent organs, such as stomach, transverse colon, left adrenal gland, and left kidney.[6,7]

TUMOR BIOLOGY

Ultimate success of any oncologic surgery depends on cancer-related survival. This specific oncological outcome is mainly driven by tumor biology, tumor margins, and adequacy of lymph node dissection.

Cystic Pancreatic Neoplasms

Most cystic neoplasms of the pancreas are benign but range from completely benign simple cysts, serous cystadenomas, and pseudocysts to potentially premalignant mucinous cystadenomas and intraducal pappilary mucinous neoplasms (IPMNs) to malignant IPMNs and malignant mucinous cystadenocarcinomas. Large neoplasm size, presence of symptoms, rapid tumor growth, and cyst fluid carcinoembryonic antigen level greater than 200 ng/mL should prompt surgery. A crucial point in LDPs for cystic neoplasm is tumor manipulation and potential rupture, which may be under-reported.

Neuroendocrine Tumors

Pancreatic neuroendocrine tumors are frequently identified incidentally. They are rare neoplasms with an incidence of 1 per 100,000. Pancreatic neuroendocrine tumors can be functional or nonfunctional. They can manifest in association with an inherited syndrome, such as multiple endocrine neoplasia, or sporadically. Song and colleagues[8] evaluated 359 patients who underwent LDP; 10% had neuroendocrine tumors. Fernandez-Cruz and colleagues[9] reported 49 patients with neuroendocrine tumors; 51% had LDP and 48% had laparoscopic enucleations with negative resection margins in all malignant lesions.

Pancreatic Ductal Adenocarcinoma

Adequate lymphadenectomy provides useful staging to influence decisions regarding adjuvant chemotherapy or chemoradiation therapy. The ratio of positive to procured lymph nodes has been shown of prognostic significance. The adequacy of lymph node dissection during LDP has been under investigation. The mean number of lymph nodes harvested has been reported between 10.3 ± 8.6 and 18 ± 4.[6,8,9]

RESECTIONS

The 3 most common types of distal pancreatic resections performed for neoplastic disease are LDP, laparoscopic spleen-preserving DP, and laparoscopic tumor enucleation of the distal pancreas.

LDP is the most common laparoscopic pancreatic resection. Gagner and colleagues[10–12] published the first 8 LDPs for islet cell tumors. Recently, large series were published showing comparative perioperative results with ODP.[6] Common variations include spleen-preserving LDP with or without splenic vessels preservation, LDP with splenectomy, and the radical antegrade modular pancreatectomy.

Preoperative Considerations

If splenectomy is anticipitated, then vaccination against encapsulated bacteria (Haemophilus influenza, Streptococcus, and Meningococcus) should be given 7 to 10 days before LDP. Patients with functional pancreatic neuroendocrine tumors require physiologic status optimization before surgery. Preoperative antibiotics and deep venous thrombosis prophylaxis are provided according to Surgical Care Improvement Project guidelines.[13]

Positioning of the Patient, Operator, and Trocars

Patients are placed in the right lateral decubitus position using beanbags or large gel rolls. This position allows gravity to play a retractor role during the mobilization. A nasogastric tube and a Foley catheter are usually placed after anesthesia induction.

The operating surgeon and the second assistant stand to the right of the patient, and the first assistant with the scrub nurse stand on the left side of the patient.

Pneumoperitoneum is established via open technique (through perimumbilical incision with 12-mm trocar under direct vision) or closed technique (Veress needle in the left upper quadrant). Abdominal pressure is maintained at 15 mm Hg by insufflation of carbon dioxide. Four trocars, 2 5-mm trocars (1 in the left flank and 2 in the epigastrium) and 2 12-mm trocars (1 in the perimumbilical region for the scope and 1 in the midclavicular line at the same level of the umbilicus), allow the procedure to progress. An additional 5-mm subxiphoid trocar is occasionally added to help in retracting the left lobe of the liver (Nathanson retractor). Surgeons should triangulate their trocars around the body/tail of the pancreas with at least 5 cm distance that allows sufficient range of motion.[14]

LAPAROSCOPIC DISTAL PANCREATECTOMY WITH EN BLOC SPLENECTOMY

Several technical variations have been described in the literature based on surgeon preference. The authors prefer the following technique.

Lesser Sac Exposure and Splenic Flexure Mobilization

After exploring the abdominal cavity for any metastases, the gastrocolic ligament is divided using LigaSure (Valleylab, Boulder, CO, USA) to open the lesser sac and to expose the plane between the posterior wall of the stomach and the body/tail of the pancreas. Short gastric vessels are divided using LigaSure to the most cephalad short gastric vessels.[15] The stomach is reflected cephalad, exposing the pancreas. The plane between the posterior stomach and the anterior surface of the pancreas is easy to develop. A laparoscopic intraoperative ultrasound probe introduced through the 12-mm trocar is helpful in selected cases for further localization. It is important in this step to place patients in reverse Trendelenburg position to allow gravity to drop the greater omentum. Care must be taken to avoid injury to the right gastroepiploic vessels and to avoid contact with gastric wall (Fig. 1).

The splenic flexure is mobilized by dividing the splenocolic ligament using LigaSure. This exposes the tail of the pancreas and the inferior pole of the spleen. The colon is reflected medially and the white line of Toldt is divided to develop adequate posterior plane for mobilization of the pancreas in the retroperitoneum. This plane is avascular separating the mesocolon form the Gerota fascia. Splenic attachments to the diaphragm should not be divided to prevent the spleen from flopping in the operative field.

Pancreatic Mobilization

The inferior border of the pancreas is dissected out and a window is created below the pancreatic edge developing a vascular posterior plane between the pancreas and the retroperitoneum. The splenic vein small branches are divided using LigaSure until the posterior surface of the pancreas is fully visualized. The dissection is carried from lateral to medial past the target lesion. The inferior mesenteric vein is identified along the inferior edge of the pancreas. Care must be taken in this step to avoid injury to the retroperitoneal structures, such as the kidney and adrenal gland. Surgeons should maintain a horizontal place during dissection (for subtotal resections, the specimen includes neck, body, tail, and the plane developed behind the pancreas is at the level of the neck).[16]

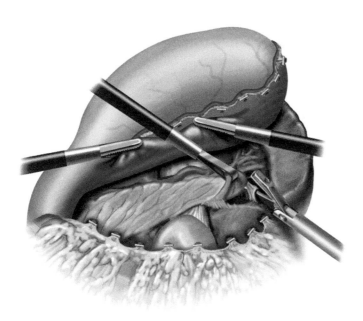

Fig. 1. The dissection is continued by creating a window below the pancreatic edge and by developing a posterior plane between the pancreas and the retroperitoneum. (*Reprinted from* Jones DB, Maithel SK, Schneider BE. Atlas of minimally invasive surgery. Woodbury (CT): Cine-Med, Inc; 2006; with permission. Copyright of the book and illustrations are retained by Cine-Med, Inc.)

Pancreatic Transection and Division of the Splenic Vein and Artery

After confirming the site of division, the pancreas is retracted superiorly and anteriorly and the dissection is continued caudal to cephalad exposing the splenic vein. A finger-type dissection may be useful.

The splenic artery is clearly identified and dissected along the superior border of the pancreas. The splenic vein is exposed again posterior to the artery. Splenic artery and vein may be divided en bloc with pancreatic parenchyma unless the pancreatic parenchyma is close to the celiac trunk, in which case the artery is better divided separately.

An articulated rotational endoscopic linear stapler with various thicknesses (staple height, 3.5–4.2 mm) is used to divide the pancreas. In selected cases, the authors apply small titanium clips or fibrin glue (Tisseel, Baxter, Deerfield, Illinois) along the staple line to control bleeding. It is not necessary to completely transect the pancreas with 1 staple firing (**Fig. 2**). In selected cases, a partial resection facilitates better exposure of the superior edge and the splenic artery for later division. The splenic artery and vein should be clearly identified and divided with linear stapler, taking care not to compromise arteries originating from the celiac trunk. The authors usually use a 45-mm or 60-mm linear stapler, which is placed through the left-sided midclavicular port to allow a direct approach to the pancreas (**Fig. 3**). In selected cases, the authors transect the splenic artery and vein with the linear stapler before the parenchymal transection. If the splenic vessels were transected proximally, they are transected again at the hilum. An extended lymphadenectomy of the celiac trunk is performed if needed by dividing the attachment of the superior edge of the pancreas to the celiac trunk. Particular care is taken to identify and individually ligate the main pancreatic duct (ultrasound may be useful in selected cases). Once the pancreas and splenic vessels

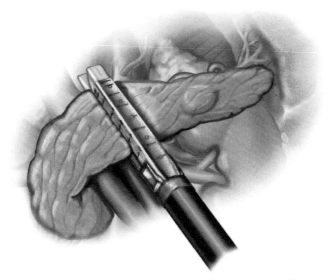

Fig. 2. An articulated rotational endoscopic linear stapler with various thicknesses is usually used depending on the thickness of the pancreatic tissue. (*Reprinted from* Jones DB, Maithel SK, Schneider BE. Atlas of minimally invasive surgery. Woodbury (CT): Cine-Med, Inc; 2006; with permission. Copyright of the book and illustrations are retained by Cine-Med, Inc.)

are completely divided, the dissection is continued along the superior edge of the spleen medial to lateral by retracting the pancreas inferiorly to expose any attachment to the retroperitoneum. In a posterior radical antegrade modular pancreatosplenectomy, the left adrenal gland and Gerota fascia are readily exposed. The spleen is freed

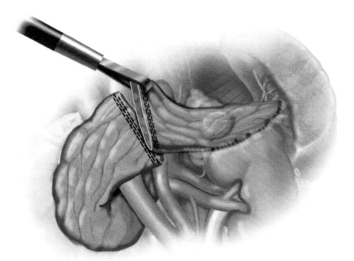

Fig. 3. The dissection is continued along the superior edge of the spleen medial to lateral by retracting the pancreas inferiorly to expose any attachment to the retroperitoneum. (*Reprinted from* Jones DB, Maithel SK, Schneider BE. Atlas of minimally invasive surgery. Woodbury (CT): Cine-Med, Inc; 2006; with permission. Copyright of the book and illustrations are retained by Cine-Med, Inc.)

of its posterior, lateral, and superior attachments. Some surgeons prefer lateral to medial dissection; pancreatic dissection starts laterally by retracting the tail of the pancreas anteriorly and medially, dividing splenic vessels branches to the pancreas. Dissection is continued medially toward the point of transection. Hand-assisted LDP may bear some advantages in selected cases involving dense adhesions, obesity, and large tumors.

Specimen Removal, Drain Placement, and Closure

The specimen is placed in an entrapment sac, which can be a frustrating step of the operation where gravity can help, and removed through the umbilical port. If the LDP is done for neoplasm, the proximal pancreatic margin should be marked and sent for frozen section. Pathologic confirmation of neuroendocrine tumor in the specimen is also a necessity and should be sent for frozen section.

A closed suction drain is placed in the left upper quadrant close to the pancreatic stump and brought out through the 5-mm trocar site. All fascial incisions greater than 10 mm should be closed.

Conversion to Open Distal Pancreatectomy

Surgeons should be as comfortable performing ODP as performing LDP. In a collective review performed in 2009, it was reported that among the 806 patients who underwent LDP, 9.2% of the patients required conversion to an open procedure. The most common indications were bleeding, adhesions, and malignancy.[7] Further studies are needed to address the effect of surgeon volume on conversion rate. An open approach is usually performed through a left subcostal incision or through upper midline. Opening the lesser sac, division of the short gastric vessels and mobilization of the splenic flexure and inferior border of the pancreas are then performed. After identifying the lesion, the pancreatic parenchyma is transected. The splenic artery and vein are isolated and ligated before or after, depending on surgeon preference.

Spleen-Preserving Distal Pancreatectomy

There are 2 described techniques to preserve the spleen in LDP. After entering the lesser sac, the pancreas is dissected off the splenic vessels. The small branches of splenic artery and vein are divided using a sealing instrument starting near the presumed line of pancreatic division toward the splenic hilum. The tail of the pancreas is fully mobilized, avoiding any injury to the splenic vessels, splenic parenchyma, or pancreatic parenchyma. In the Warshaw technique, once the splenic artery or vein is ligated, short gastric vessels are preserved to spare the blood supply to the spleen.[17]

It is the authors' preference to preserve the splenic artery and vein to maintain the immunologic function of the spleen.

Pancreatic Enucleation (Body/Tail)

There are several small series reporting laparoscopic enucleation for insulinoma (the most common functional pancreatic endocrine tumor). In this approach, the tumor is enucleated and the surrounding pancreatic parenchyma is preserved. Small tumors with indolent behavior, located away from the main pancreatic duct, are mostly suitable for laparoscopic enucleation using laparoscopic ultrasound. As with LDPs, pancreatic fistula remains an issue (**Box 1**).

> **Box 1**
> **Technical considerations for LDP**
>
> 1. Surgeons should save the inferior mesenteric vein (located lateral to the ligament of Treitz at the midportion of the body of the pancreas) as it courses to join the splenic vein.
> 2. An extra hand port or subxiphoid liver retractor port could facilitate exposure in selected cases with inadequate exposure.
> 3. If varices are encountered during dissection of the splenic vessels, it is recommended to use clips for vessel control.
> 4. Pancreatic surgeons should benefit from laparoscopic ultrasound, especially in small tumors.

POSTOPERATIVE CARE
Morbidities and Mortality

LDP is a safe procedure with a low mortality rate (0.25%) but complications range from 30% to 40%. Pancreatic-related complications include pancreatic fistula, pancreatic abscess, pancreatic pseudocyst, pancreatitis, and intra-abdominal fluid collection. Pulmonary complications include pleural complications, pneumonia, and pulmonary embolism. Other morbidities are surgical site infections, postoperative bleeding, and splenic complications (mostly splenic infarct).[18–20]

Regarding risk factors, Weber and colleagues[21] analyzed 219 patients undergoing LDP over 8 years from 9 academic medical centers to assess risk factors for perioperative complications. Thirty-day morbidity and mortality were 39% and 0, respectively. Major complications occurred in 11%. Pancreatic fistulae were detected in 23%, with clinically important fistulae (grade B/C) seen in 10%. A complication risk score, consisting of 1 point each for body mass index greater than 27, pancreatic specimen length greater than 8 cm, or excess body mass index lost greater than 150 mL, predicted an increased risk of complications, including pancreatic fistulae. The risk score should be used in operative planning and risk assessment. A review of 2322 patients who underwent DP using the American College of Surgeons National Surgical Quality Improvement Program reported 30-day complication and mortality rates of 28.1% and 1.2%, respectively. Serious complications were found in 22.2%; the most common included sepsis (8.7%), surgical site infection (5.9%), and pneumonia (4.7%). Risk factors associated with morbidity included male gender, body mass index greater than 30, smoking, steroid use, neurologic disease, hypoalbunemia, elevated creatinine, systemic inflammatory response syndrome/sepsis, and thrombocytosis. Preoperative factors associated with 30-day mortality included esophageal varices, neurologic disease, dependent functional status, recent weight loss, elevated alkaline phosphatase, and elevated blood urea nitrogen. Operative risk factors for both morbidity and mortality included intraoperative transfusion requirement ($\geq$3 units) and prolonged operative time (>6 hours).[22]

Management of the Pancreatic Stump

Pancreatic fistula is a common complication after LDP and is defined as a concentration of drain amylase 5 times greater than the upper limit of normal in serum and a drain of more than 30 mL at 5 days or longer after surgery (Sarr criteria).

According to the 2005 ISGPF,[13] pancreatic fistula is defined as output via an operatively placed drain (or a subsequently placed percutaneous drain) of any measurable volume of drain fluid on or after postoperative day 3, with an amylase content greater than 3 times the upper normal serum value; each pancreatic fistula was classified as grade A, B, or C. The clinical manifestations, as defined by ISGPF, range from asymptomatic fluid drainage in closed suction drains to life-threatening sepsis requiring surgical intervention: "Output via an operatively placed drain (or a subsequently placed, percutaneous drain) of any measurable volume of drain fluid on or after postoperative day 3, with an amylase content greater than 3 times the upper normal value serum level"[13] (**Box 2**).

Several trials have investigated methods of resolving the ongoing debate about prevention of pancreatic fistula in LDP. Trials included tailored application of different linear stapler thickness depending on the quality of the pancreatic parenchyma with or without staple line reinforcement, using low-intensity electrocautery on the stump, application of small titanium clips and/or application of fibrin glue, covering the pancreatic stump with omentum and gastric wall after placing closed suction drain and encouraging patients to stay in a semi–left-lateral position on the first postoperative day, main duct suture ligation, oversewing of the pancreatic stump, ultrasound coagulation, octreotide administration, pancreaticoenteric anastomosis, fixation of the tip of a peripancreatic drain with a loose loop, jejunal seromuscular or gastricserosal patches, fixation of the tip of a peripancreatic drain for effective drainage after DP, a recent novel technique with duct-to-mucosa pancreaticogastrostomy, or various combinations of these techniques. Use of the LigaSure sealing device for transection of the pancreas is under investigation on animal models by a group in Germany.[23–27]

Duct-to-mucosa pancreaticogastrostomy has been described by Sudo and colleagues[26] in 21 patients who underwent DP. Morbidity was 5% with no mortality. The postoperative pancreatic fistula rate of clinically relevant grade B or grade C fistulae was 0%, although grade A fistula rate was 29%.

Other limited studies have shown the advantage of pancreaticoenteric anastomosis for preventing pancreatic fistulae after DP. In a prospective trial, Wagner and colleagues[28] performed an anastomosis of the pancreatic stump into a jejunal Roux-en-Y limb by a single-layer suture after DP in 23 patients. The Roux-en-Y anastomosis was associated with no postoperative clinical pancreatic fistulae compared with the traditional hand-sewn closure method after which fistulae developed in 20% of cases. Kleef and colleagues[29] reported that in a large retrospective study in 302 consecutive distal pancreatectomies, the pancreatic fistula rate after various types of closure, including pancreaticojejunal anastomosis (n = 24), seromuscular

---

Box 2
Clinical grading of pancreatic fistula according to the International Study Group on Pancreatic Fistula definition

Grade A

　Transient fistula with no clinical effect

Grade B

　Required change in management (eg, partial or total parenteral nutrition, interventional drainage, antibiotics, somatostatin analogs, extended hospital stay, or readmission)

Grade C

　Major change in clinical management (eg, total parenteral nutrition, intravenous antibiotics, somatostatin analogs, sepsis, organ dysfunction, surgical intervention, revision of anastomosis, or delay in hospital discharge)

patch (n = 36), stapler (n = 145), and suture (n = 97), were 0%, 8.3%, 15.9%, and 9.3%, respectively. Pancreaticogastrostomy after DP has benefits compared with Roux-en-Y pancreaticojejunostomy, including a single anastomosis, potentially shorter surgical times, and the preservation of gastrointestinal tract integrity. Further randomized clinical trials comparing these methods with standard procedures are required to confirm their actual efficacy, taking into consideration increasing the complexity of the operation.

Identification and selective ligation of the main pancreatic duct remain a challenging step in the laparoscopic approach and is considered one of the steps at the authors' institution. Bilimoria and colleagues[30] performed an analysis of 126 patients over 9 years with pancreatic fistula rate of 9.6% in the 74 cases of duct ligation and 34% in the 53 cases without duct ligation (P<.001). They concluded that the absence of selective ligation of the main pancreatic duct was the only factor that maintained association with increased risk of pancreatic fistula.

Stapling has been suggested to increase fistula rate in a study by Reeh and colleagues,[17] in which they performed 283 LDPs using 3 different techniques with stapler resulting in significantly higher morbidity (pancreatic fistula) in comparison with hand-sewn anastomosis and pancreaticojejunostomy, whereas, Jimenez and colleagues[27] favored stapling and reinforcement in their series and demonstrated that staple line reinforcement reduces pancreatic fistula rate after DP. Further validation is needed in randomized controlled trials.

The multi-institutional DISPACT trial, a randomized controlled trial done in 21 European hospitals, was designed to assess the effect of stapler versus hand-sewn closure on formation of postoperative pancreatic fistula after DP. In 450 patients, the pancreatic fistula rate was 32% in the stapler group versus 28% in the hand-sewn group (P = .56). Both stapler and hand-sewn closure were equally safe after DP. The DISPACT trial did not show a reduction in postoperative pancreatic fistula and mortality up to postoperative day 7 by stapler resection and closure compared with scalpel resection and hand-sewn closure of the pancreatic remnant for DP.[25]

ROBOTIC DISTAL PANCREATECTOMY

For the past 10 years, robotic surgery has been slowly gaining popularity within the world of minimally invasive surgery. Robotic distal pancreatectomy (RDP) is limited by the lack of data regarding long-term oncologic outcome and a steep learning curve. The few case series in RDP are optimistic, advocating that those limited benefits are important enough to take the challenge of learning robotic procedures.[31–33]

Kang and colleagues[32] in Seoul reviewed 45 patients who underwent LDP (25 patients) or RDP (20 patients) for benign and borderline malignant lesions. They found that RDP was superior to LDP in spleen preservation but inferior with regard to cost and length of procedure, whereas Zureikat and colleagues[34] recently demonstrated in their case series of 30 patients that robotic pancreatic procedures can be done safely in a high-volume pancreatic tertiary center with perioperative outcomes comparable to those of ODP.

DISCUSSION

LDP is reserved for well-trained surgeons in advanced laparoscopic surgery. Few surgeons have expertise in LDPs. Current literature suggest that it is overall feasible, safe, and beneficial with regard to faster return to normal activities, reduced postoperative pain, reduced hospital stay, and better scar scores.[35,36] With a lack of randomized controlled trials, however, the role and oncologic safety of LDP for pancreatic cancer remain unknown.

LDP has been mostly used for benign pancreatic lesions (serous cystic neoplasm) and low-grade malignant lesions (mucinous cystic neoplasms and IPMNs). The oncologic safety (completeness of the resection, nodal evaluation, and survival) of LDP remains, however, under investigation and limited. Surgeons considering LDP must confirm that they can achieve adequate clear margins and lymph node dissection. All existing reports addressing LDP are retrospective and have small numbers.

The role of splenic preservation remains controversial, but overall it has been reported more frequently with LDP than with ODP. Butturini and colleagues[37]showed the rate of splenic preservation was significantly higher in an LDP group (44.2) than an ODP (11%) group. DiNorica and colleagues,[38] in their 360 distal pancreatectomies results comparing ODP and LDP, concluded that both have comparable rates of splenic preservation. During LDP, surgeons aim to preserve the spleen, unless the tumor is close to the splenic hilum or ischemia is noticed after dividing the splenic vessels (Warshaw technique) but only if malignancy is excluded. More controlled studies are needed to compare LDP with ODP in malignant pancreatic lesions. Alvise and colleagues[18] performed a retrospective analysis of 10 patients who underwent LDP for solid pseudopapillary tumors; 50% underwent LDP with en bloc splenectomy and 50% underwent spleen-preserving LDP (3 with splenic vessel preservation and 2 with Warshaw technique). After a median follow-up of 47 (5–98 range) months, all patients were alive and disease-free. Another study from Song and colleagues[8] in Seoul addressed perioperative outcomes for 359 patients who underwent LDP. Of these, 90% had benign or low-grade malignant neoplasms and 10% had malignancies. Of these, 49.6% had spleen-preserving LDP (41.8% SP-LDP without splenic vessels ligation and 7.8% SP-LDP with splenic vessel ligation). Overall, the complications rate after LDP was 12% (including pancreatic fistula, 7%). Cruz and colleagues[39] in Barcelona studied 82 patients; 52 had their spleens preserved with or without splenic vessels preservation and they concluded that overall complications were higher in the splenic preservation group. DiNorica and colleagues[38] suggested no difference in clinical outcomes between spleen-preserving DP and DP with splenectomy with regard to morbidity, pancreatic fistula, and hospital length of stay. The study included a confounding bias, which was performing DP with selective spleen preservation when oncologically appropriate.

In the absence of level 1 data demonstrating clear benefit, LDP with spleen preservation can be considered a matter of surgical preference and is not recommended in cases of suspected or confirmed adenocarcinoma of the body/tail of the pancreas or in cases of pancreatic endocrine tumors in which splenic vessels are encased.

Borja-Cacho and colleagues[7] analyzed the oncologic appropriateness of LDP for pancreatic cancer in their systematic review of the literature and concluded that it remains unknown. Despite the willingness of several investigators to perform LDP in the face of known malignancy, there is a lack of standard reporting of oncologic outcomes. Kooby and colleagues[40,41] reported as well that LDP provides similar short-term and long-term oncologic outcomes compared with OPD for pancreatic ductal adenocarcinoma, according to a multicenter analysis. Because of the lack of level 1 data on LDP for cancer, it is safe to report that current evidence is insufficient to recommend or discourage LDP for patients with pancreatic adenocarcinoma or mucinous cystadenocarcinoma.

Single-institutional and multi-institutional reports exist comparing the safety and efficacy of LDP and ODP. These data suggest that the cosmetic results of laparoscopic approach are superior to those of ODP. LDP has a shorter length of stay, less pain, earlier return to normal bowel function and diet, and similar incidence in pancreatic fistula and may be associated with reduced blood loss and greater likelihood of splenic preservation.

DiNorica and colleagues[38] concluded that both OPD and LDP have comparable rates of splenic preservation, pancreatic fistula, and mortality. LDP had lower blood loss and smaller tumor size. LDP had fewer complications overall as well as shorter hospital stays. Similar results were found in a meta-analysis done by Nigri and colleagues[19] in reviewing 10 studies, including 349 LDPs and 380 ODPs.

Although the length of procedures are reported as significantly longer for LDP in comparison with ODP in few retrospective studies, length of procedures for LDP is reduced when laparoscopic surgeons with adequate experience perform operations. Song and colleagues[8] found that operative time decreased as surgeons' experience increased and, after 20 LDPs, the operative time for LDP approached those (190–226 minutes) for ODP.

Conversion has been reported caused by difficult exposure, invasion of surgical margin, bleeding, and inability to localize small pancreatic tumors. Ammori and Ayiomamitis[35] reported, in their review of the literature, a conversion rate of 11.5%. In a multi-institution study of 667 patients after LPDs, there was a significance decrease in blood loss and hospital stay in comparison with ODPs. Similar results were reported by Jayaraman and colleagues[36] at the Memorial Sloan–Kettering Cancer Center in their review of 343 DPs.

Lastly, LDP is a safe procedure with a low mortality rate and significant morbidities of 30% to 40%, including pancreatic fistula (16.8%), which is similar to that in ODP performed at a high-volume center. Different definitions of pancreatic fistula might underestimate that complication rate. It is important in the future reporting to follow the standard ISGPF guidelines. The volume-to-outcomes relationship for LDP requires additional investigation. Reports of LDP in children demonstrate the safety and efficacy in the pediatric population.[42]

SUMMARY

There has been a tremendous growth in the number of reports concerning LDP during the past 5 years. Greater emphasis is applied to patient outcomes (pancreatic fistula, morbidities, and hospital stay). With the recently published noninferior cancer-related outcomes data, the time is potentially right for a randomized controlled trial to address the true value of LDP for cancer. The greatest limitation to this potential trial is the number of available cases of patients with body and tail adenocarcinoma; a trial requires enrollment of more than 1000 patients to prove noninferiority of either approach and likely requires the participation of every tertiary medical center in the United states. Ideally, pancreatic surgeons should follow the example set by the authors' colorectal colleagues and design prospective, multicenter, randomized trials comparing LDP with ODP for malignancies.

In conclusion, LDP is a safe procedure with a morbidity rate that is comparable with that of ODP and should be performed by experienced, high-volume surgeons. Laparoscopic approach should be offered for benign lesions in the body/tail of the pancreas. Pancreatic surgeons should report their outcomes diligently (resection margin, lymph node count, and morbidity rate, including pancreatic fistula) and follow the recommendations of the ISGPF.

REFERENCES

1. Kang CM, Kim DH, Lee WJ. Ten years of experience of experience with resection of left-sided pancreatic ductal adenocarcinoma: evolution and initial experience to a laparoscopic approach. Surg Endosc 2010;24:1533–41.
2. Briggs CD, Mann CD, Irving GR, et al. Systematic review of minimal invasive pancreatic resection. J Gastrointest Surg 2009;13:1129–37.
3. Kooby DA, Chu CK. Laparoscopic management of pancreatic malignancies. Surg Clin North Am 2010;90(2):427–46 Review.
4. Lenoon AM, Newman N, Makary MA, et al. EUS-guided tattooing before laparoscopic distal resection (with video). Gastrointest Endosc 2010;72(5):1089–94.
5. Newman NA, Lennon AM, Edil BH, et al. Preoperative endoscopic tattooing of pancreatic body and tail lesions decreases operative time for laparoscopic distal pancreatectomy. Surgery 2010;148(2):371–7.
6. Kooby DA, Hawkinds WG, Schmidt CM, et al. A multicenter analysis of distal pancreatectomy for adenocarcinoma: is laparoscopic resection appropriate? J Am Coll Surg 2010;210(5):779–85.
7. Borja-Cacho D, Al-Refaie W, Vickers S, et al. Laparoscopic distal pancreatectomy. J Am Coll Surg 2009;209(6):758–65.
8. Song KB, Kim SC, Park JB, et al. Single-center experience of laparoscopic left pancreatic resection in 359 consecutive patients: changing the surgical paradigm of left pancreatic resection. Surg Endosc 2011;10:3364–72.
9. Fernandez-Cruz L, Blanco L, Cosa R, et al. Is laparoscopic resection adequate in patients with neuroendocrine pancreatic tumors? World J Surg 2008;32(5):904–17.
10. Gagner M, Pomp A, Herrera MF. Early experience with laparoscopic resections of islet cell tumors. Surgery 1996;120(6):1051–4.
11. Gagner M. Pioneers in laparoscopic solid organ surgery. Surg Endosc 2003;17:1853–4.
12. Gagner M, Palermo M. Laparoscopic Whipple procedure: review of the literature. J Hepatobiliary Pancreat Surg 2009;16:726–30.
13. Jones DB, Maithel SK, Schneider BE. Atlas of minimally invasive surgery. 1st edition. Woodbury (CT): Cine-Med, Inc; 2006. p. 406–29.
14. Hartwig W, Duckheim M, Strobel O, et al. Ligasure for pancreatic sealing during distal pancreatectomy. World J Surg 2010;34:1066–70.
15. Pham TH, Gilbert EW, The SH, et al. Distal pancreatic resection chapter. In: Vernon A, editor. Atlas of minimally invasive surgical techniques. St Louis (MO): Elsevier; 2012.
16. Warshaw AL. Conservation of the spleen with distal pancreatectomy. Arch Surg 1988;123:550–3.
17. Reeh M, Nentwich MF, Bogoevski D, et al. High surgical morbidity following distal pancreatectomy: still an unsolved problem. World J Surg 2011;35:1110–7.
18. Alvise C, Giovanni B, Desoina D, et al. Laparoscopic Pancreatectomy for solid pseudo-papillary tumor of the pancreas is a suitable technique; our experience with long-term follow-up and review of the literature. Ann Surg Oncol 2011;18(2):352–7.
19. Nigri GR, Roseman AS, Petrucciani N, et al. Metaanalysis of trials comparing minimally invasive and open pancreatectomies. Surg Endosc 2011;25(5):1642–51.
20. Weber SM, Cho CS, Merchant N, et al. Laparoscopic left pancreatectomy: complication risk score correlates with morbididty and risk for pancreatic fistula. Ann Surg Oncol 2009;16:2825–33.

21. Kelly KJ, Greenblatt DY, Wan Y, et al. Risk stratification for distal pancreatectomy utilizing ACS-NSQIP: preoperative factors predict morbidity and mortality. J Gastrointest Surg 2011;15:250–61.

22. Bassi C, Dervenis C, Butturini G, et al. Postoperative pancreatic fistula: an international study group (ISGPF) definition. Surgery 2005;138(1):8–13.

23. Sugiyama M, Suzuki Y, Nobutsugu A, et al. Secure placement of a peripancreatic drain after a distal pancreatectomy. Am J Surg 2010;199:178–82.

24. Velanovich V. The use of tissue sealant to prevent fistula formation after laparoscopic distal pancreatectomy. Surg Endosc 2007;21:1222.

25. Diener MK, Seiler CM, Rossion I, et al. Efficacy of stapler versus hand-sewn closure after distal pancreatectomy (DISPACT): a randomized, controlled multicentre trial. Lancet 2011;377:1514–22.

26. Sudo T, Murakami Y, Uemura K, et al. Dital pancreatectomy with duct-to-mucosa pancreaticogastrostomy: a novel technique for preventing postoperative pancreatic fistula. Am J Surg 2011;202:77–81.

27. Jiminez RE, Mavanur A, Macaulay WP. Staple line reinforcement reduces postoperative pancreatic stump leak after distal pancreatectomy. J Gastrointest Surg 2007;11(3):345–9.

28. Wagner M, Gloor B, Mabuhl M, et al. Roux-en-Y drainage of the pancreatic stump decreases pancreatic fistula after distal pancreatic resection. J Gastrointest Surg 2007;11(3):303–8.

29. Kleeff J, Diener MK, Z'graggen K, et al. Distal pancreatectomy: risk factors for surgical failure in 302 consecutive cases. Ann Surg 2007;245(4):573–82.

30. Bilimoria M, Cormier J, Mun Y, et al. Pancreatic leak after left pancreatectomy is reduced following main pancreatic duct ligation. Br J Surg 2003;90(2):190–6.

31. Ntourakis D, Marzano E, Penza P, et al. Robotic distal splenopancreatectomy: bridging the gap between pancreatic and minimal access surgery. J Gastrointest Surg 2010;14:1326–30.

32. Kang CM, Kim DH, Lee WJ, et al. Conventional laparoscopic and robot-assisted spleen-preserving pancreatectomy: does da Vinci have clinical advantages? Surg Endosc 2011;25:2004–9.

33. Kang CM, Choi SH, Hwang HK, et al. Minimally invasive (laparoscopic and robot-assisted) approach for solid pseudopapillary tumor of the distal pancreas: a single-center experience. J Hepatobiliary Pancreat Sci 2011;18:87–93.

34. Zureikat AH, Nguyen KT, Bartlett DL, et al. Robotic-assisted major pancreatic resection and reconstruction. Arch Surg 2011;146(3):256–61.

35. Ammori BJ, Ayiomamitis GD. Laparoscopic pancreaticoduodenectomy and distal pancreatectomy: a UK experience and a systematic review of the literature. Surg Endosc 2011;25:2084–99.

36. Jayaraman S, Gnonen M, Brennan M, et al. Laparoscopic distal pancreatectomy: evolution of technique at a single institution. J Am Coll Surg 2010;211(4):503–9.

37. Butturini G, Partelli S, Crippa S, et al. Perioperative and long-term results after left pancreatectomy: a single-institution, non-randomized, comparative study between open and laparoscopic approach. Surg Endosc 2011;25:2871–8.

38. DiNorcia J, Schrope BA, Lee MK, et al. Laparoscopic distal pancreatectomy offers shorter hospital stays with fewer complications. J Gastrointest Surg 2010;14:1804–12.

39. Fernández-Cruz L, Cosa R, Blanco L, et al. Curative laparoscopic resection for pancreatic neoplasms: a critical analysis from a single institution. J Gastrointest Surg 2007;11(12):1607.

40. Kooby DA, Gillespie T, Bentrem D, et al. Left-sided pancreatectomy: a multi-center comparison of laparoscopic and open approaches. Ann Surg 2008; 248:438–46.
41. Finan KR, Cannon EE, Kim EJ, et al. Laparoscopic and open distal pancreatectomy: a comparison of outcomes. Am Surg 2009;75:671–9 [discussion: 679–80].
42. Melotti G, Cavallini A, Butturini G, et al. Laparoscopic distal pancreatectomy in childen: case report and review of the literature. Ann Surg Oncol 2007;14(3): 1065–9.

Laparoscopic Resection of the Liver for Cancer

Emily Winslow, MD[a],*, William G. Hawkins, MD[b]

KEYWORDS

- Laparoscopy • Liver Resection • Hepatic Resection • Metastatic colorectal cancer
- Hepatocellular carcinoma

KEY POINTS

- Laparoscopic hepatic resection has been most widely applied to patients with solitary and symptomatic benign tumors.
- Tumors in the segments II, III, IVb, V, and VI are more assessable for laparoscopic resection, whereas those in segments VII, VIII, and IVa are the most difficult to resect laparoscopically.
- Studies of carefully selected patients to date suggest less blood loss for laparoscopic hepatic resections, but concern over the rare but not infrequently reported occurrence of significant intraoperative hemorrhage from vascular injuries continues to warrant careful study.
- For selected patients with a solitary hepatocellular carcinoma, laparoscopic hepatic resection should be considered and seems to be associated with some advantages.
- For patients with metastatic colorectal cancer, laparoscopic hepatic resection should only be applied in cases that have adequate room between the tumor and the transaction plane to ensure an adequate margin.
- Detailed preoperative imaging and liberal use of intraoperative ultrasound are helpful adjuncts for assessing the residual hepatic parenchyma, especially when a hand-port device is not used.
- Ongoing randomized clinical trials coming open to laparoscopic resection of both metastatic colorectal lesions and hepatocellular carcinomas will certainly enhance the current understanding of the role of laparoscopic hepatic resection for cancer.

HISTORY OF LAPAROSCOPIC HEPATIC RESECTIONS

Gagner and colleagues[1] is credited with reporting the first laparoscopic hepatic resection in 1992. In an abstract presented at the Annual Meeting of the Society of American

[a] Hepatopancreaticobiliary Surgery, Division of General Surgery, Department of Surgery, University of Wisconsin School of Medicine and Public Health, K4/749 CSC 600 Highland Avenue, Madison, WI 53792-7375, USA; [b] Section of Hepatobiliary, Pancreatic and Gastrointestinal Surgery, Department of Surgery, Washington University School of Medicine, 660 South Euclid Avenue, Campus Box 8109, St. Louis, MO 63110, USA
* Corresponding author.
E-mail address: winslow@surgery.wisc.edu

Surg Oncol Clin N Am 22 (2013) 75–89
http://dx.doi.org/10.1016/j.soc.2012.08.005
surgonc.theclinics.com

Gastrointestinal and Endoscopic Surgeons, he described 2 patients. The first was a young woman with a 6-cm lesion in segment VI, which was thought to be an adenoma, but after she underwent a laparoscopic wedge resection, it was found instead to be focal nodular hyperplasia. The second patient had metastatic colorectal cancer, and a wedge resection in segment V was undertaken. Both specimens were removed transvaginally and the patients were discharged within 4 days postoperatively.

The following year, the first report of a laparoscopic anatomic hepatic resection was published by Azagra and colleagues,[2] who described a left lateral sectionectomy (resection of segments II and III) for a symptomatic hepatic adenoma. Not until 4 years later in 1997 was the first major anatomic hepatic resection reported. Huscher and colleagues[3] reported a series of 20 patients in which 6 patients underwent left hemihepatectomy, 5 underwent right hemihepatectomies, and 3 had central hepatectomies.

Although the Italian group had reported the abovementioned series of complex resections 3 years prior, a seminal publication in 2000 by Cherqui and colleagues[4] is often credited as being the first reported series of laparoscopic hepatic resections. The group from the Hopital Henri Mondor in Paris reported 30 patients who largely underwent laparoscopic segmentectomies. This publication in the *Annals of Surgery* seemed to ignite the spark in many hepatic surgeons, and the laparoscopic approach to hepatic resections began to be used more widely. These authors chose to use laparoscopic approaches on patients with hepatocellular carcinoma (HCC), and excluded any patients with colorectal metastases.

EVOLUTION OF LAPAROSCOPIC HEPATIC RESECTIONS

Between 1997 and 2007, many case series of laparoscopic liver resections were published, but most of these included fewer than 30 patients. Things changed rapidly, however, in 2007 when a series of 300 laparoscopic liver resections was presented by Koffron and colleagues[5] from Northwestern University at the American Surgical Association's Annual Meeting. This report was greeted with much skepticism, as reflected by the discussants questioning the applicability of the procedure to patients with cancer, its safety, and the method through which the technique could be disseminated safely. Despite the concern from senior surgeons, the following year at the same meeting, the group from Cincinnati presented a series of 500 minimally invasive hepatic procedures, which included 253 patients who underwent laparoscopic hepatic resection.[6]

Although these 2 series are still the largest single-center experiences published, many other groups began to publish their experience with laparoscopic liver resection. By the end of 2008, reports of nearly 3000 patients had been published in the worldwide literature. In a review of this literature, nearly half of the cases were undertaken for hepatic malignancies.[7] Of those with malignant indications for resection, 52% had HCC, 35% had metastatic colorectal cancer, and 13% had other malignancies. Further, the trend was that of an exponentially increasing number of patients undergoing laparoscopic resections each year, with the fraction of those with malignant indications rapidly increasing.

THE LOUISVILLE STATEMENT

In 2008, Buell's[8] group for the University of Louisville coordinated an international consensus conference to discuss the major issues in laparoscopic liver surgery. Approximately 300 attendees were present and a variety of important topics were addressed, some of which are summarized in the following list.

1. The terms for a variety of resection types that had emerged were more clearly defined. These included pure laparoscopy, hand-assisted laparoscopy, and the hybrid technique. The latter refers to laparoscopic mobilization and dissection, but standard open parenchymal transection via a small open incision.
2. The concern for patient safety was emphasized by the conclusion stating that safety could be compromised by too rapid a dissemination of the procedure, inadequate training, and lack of established standards. However, the group concluded that the evidence available at the time could not be assessed rigorously to address the issues of patient safety.
3. The best indications for a laparoscopic approach were thought to be solitary tumors smaller than 5 cm located in hepatic segments II through VI. The group concluded that laparoscopic resection of the left lateral section (segments II and III) should be the standard of care.
4. The group emphasized that the indications for the resection of benign tumors of the liver should not be adapted despite the easier method of abdominal access.
5. The group advocated the development of a cooperative patient registry for all laparoscopic hepatic resections, which could be used to monitor for safety concerns and outcomes. This resource was thought to be more useful and more practical than a clinical trial, which would likely be underfunded and underpowered and have difficulty with accrual. However, this registry has also proven to be difficult because of its voluntary nature, tendency for underreporting, and the possibility of reflecting patient selection.
6. Finally, the most controversial area of the consensus conference was the application of laparoscopic techniques to hepatic resection in those with HCC and metastatic colorectal cancer.
   a. For metastatic colorectal cancer, the primary concerns discussed were those of margin status and inadequate evaluation of the remainder of the liver. The group concluded that patient selection and proper preoperative staging were critical to the use of laparoscopic liver resection in patients with metastatic colorectal cancer to avoid an increase in margin-positive resections and of unrecognized occult lesions.
   b. For HCC, the role of resection relative to ablation and transplantation was debated, but the group concluded that laparoscopic approaches could be useful in its treatment.

THE RESPONSE OF THE SURGICAL COMMUNITY

Although many surgeons facile with laparoscopic techniques were enthusiastic about the promise of laparoscopic hepatic resections, others were concerned about the potential for harm. In a letter to the editor entitled "A Serious Note of Caution," Donadon and colleagues[9] argue against several specific issues in Dr Buell's manuscript, but conclude as follows: "We are afraid that the infectious enthusiasm on laparoscopy in liver surgery may lead to the adoption of a technique indiscriminately to the detriment of an increase in morbidity and mortality, which should be reduced, making this aim the absolute priority rather than the reduction of the length of the incisions."

In a separate letter to the editor, Abdalla[10] disputes the suggestion made by Buell and colleagues that laparoscopic major hepatic resection represents an "evolution in the standard of care." He emphasizes the lack of data supporting this assertion, and asserts that no consensus exists about the general application of laparoscopic hepatic resections, particularly for patients with cancer. He contends that because high-quality data do not exist, one must be careful not to make assumptions about the procedure's safety and efficacy based on the less reliable data in the literature to that point. He cautions, "Care must be exercised drawing far-reaching conclusions from insufficient, evolving data."[10]

BOTH SIDES OF THE COIN

Clearly, laparoscopic hepatic resection has its clear proponents and those who are much less enthusiastic about its promise. **Box 1** outlines the potential advantages and disadvantages of the approach.

DIRECT COMPARISON OF LAPAROSCOPIC AND OPEN HEPATIC RESECTIONS

To address the potential advantages and disadvantages of laparoscopic hepatectomy, many authors have reported series of laparoscopic liver resections and others have reported case-matched comparison studies to open hepatic resections. Currently, no randomized data comparing these 2 approaches exist, and therefore systematic review and meta-analysis should be used to best compare these 2 techniques with the available data.

Box 1
Potential advantages and disadvantages of a laparoscopic approach to hepatic resection

Potential advantages

1. Because the access is less invasive, the physiologic insult to the patient should be a lesser magnitude, as evidenced by things like less postoperative pain and shorter hospital stays.

2. The reduction in blood loss during laparoscopic surgery should translate into fewer transfusions and potentially better immunologic and oncologic outcomes for patients.

3. The laparoscopic approach should be associated with fewer complications, and therefore a faster return to full functioning. This result should impact both the quality of life postoperatively and the ability to receive any planned adjuvant chemotherapy.

4. The laparoscopic approach will result in fewer adhesions, making repeat hepatic resections and potential future hepatic transplantation technically easier.

Potential disadvantages

1. The change in abdominal wall access may encourage surgeons to alter the indications for resection of benign lesions, and therefore patients may undergo unnecessary procedures.

2. The loss of the ability to palpate the liver bimanually and to explore the remainder of the abdominal cavity during a laparoscopic approach may increase the number of radiographically occult malignant lesions that go undiscovered during hepatic resection.

3. The inability to palpate the tumor and to appreciate its location in 3 dimensions may result in a higher margin-positivity rate for malignant lesions.

4. The risk of rare catastrophic events (eg, massive hemorrhage, air embolism), which could be dealt with during open hepatectomy but are more difficult to manage laparoscopically, may increase and compromise patient safety. Although difficult to quantitate, it seems from clinical anecdotal experience that these events are certainly underrepresented in the current literature.

5. The type of resection chosen may become dictated by the technique, rather than oncologic principles and patient safety. For example, a laparoscopic right hemihepatectomy might be chosen instead of a posterior sectionectomy for a solitary metastatic lesion in segment VII because of the difference in the difficulty of laparoscopic techniques.

The Findings of 2 Recent Meta-Analyses

Two recent reviews have been published and address many of the relevant comparisons discussed earlier. The first systematic review was published in 2011 but only included studies published before December of 2009.[11] Only English-language studies comparing open and laparoscopic hepatic resections that reported on perioperative and postoperative outcomes were included. A total of 26 studies were included, which resulted in a patient population of 1678. Laparoscopic resection was performed in 43% of these, with the remainder being open resections. The indication for resection was malignant disease in 62% of the laparoscopic group and 65% of the open group. Nearly two-thirds of the malignant cases in the laparoscopic group had HCC. The most relevant results of this meta-analysis are as follows:

- The duration of operation was significantly longer in the laparoscopic group (odds ratio [OR], 0.536; 95% CI, 0.120–0.952; $P = .012$)
- The median blood loss was less for the laparoscopic group (320 vs 483 mL; OR −1.109; SD −1.549, −0.669; $P<0.001$)
- Fewer overall complications occurred after laparoscopic hepatectomy (OR, 0.452; 95% CI, 0.345–0.590; $P<.001$). Similarly, fewer liver specific complications occurred after laparoscopic hepatectomy (OR, 0.636; 95% CI, 0.422–0.960; $P = .012$).
- Median length of hospital stay was less in the laparoscopic group (8 vs 10 days; OR, −1.109; 95% CI, −1.549 to −0.669; $P<.001$).
- No difference in the resection margin obtained was found between groups. Looking only at the studies that compared the incidence of a margin less than 1 cm, meta-analysis showed an increased incidence of close resection margins in those undergoing open hepatectomy.

A second similar meta-analysis was published in 2011 and included studies published until January of 2010.[12] Their search also included only those studies comparing open and laparoscopic hepatectomy with perioperative outcome measures specified, which resulted in 32 studies, totalling 2466 patients. Of these, 47% underwent laparoscopic resection. The key findings of this study are as follows:

- Again, the duration of operation was significantly longer in the laparoscopic group, but only by a clinically insignificant value of 14 minutes ($P = .02$).
- The blood loss in the laparoscopic group was less by 184 mL, and the number of patients needing transfusion was also less in the laparoscopic group (OR, 0.36; 95% CI, 0.23–0.74; $P>.001$).
- Fewer significant complications were noted in the laparoscopic group (OR, 0.35; 95% CI, 0.28–0.45; $P<.001$), but no significant difference was seen between the groups regarding chest, urinary, and wound infections.
- The duration of hospital stay was less in the laparoscopic group by nearly 3 days ($P<.001$).
- No significant difference in resection margins was seen between the groups.

The Limitations of These Findings

Taken together, these 2 meta-analyses suggest that the laparoscopic approach to hepatectomy may be associated with less blood loss and fewer transfusions, fewer postoperative complications, and a shorter hospital stay. Further, the laparoscopic approach does not seem to compromise margin status but may take longer to complete. Although these types of data provide a helpful summary of all the individual series published to date, there are significant limitations to their use, primarily the following:

1. The data from each study included in the analyses are no doubt affected by selection bias, because the patients were carefully selected on clinical grounds for the laparoscopic approach.
2. Significant heterogeneity is present in the studies included, which limits the ability to draw conclusions from the data.
3. Most of these studies included the learning curve of each group, and therefore the data are not necessarily generalizable to the current conditions surrounding laparoscopic hepatectomy.
4. Most of the cases included only laparoscopic wedge resection or left lateral sectionectomy, and therefore may not apply to more extensive hepatic resections.
5. More recent studies published over the past 2 years are not included and no updated meta-analysis is yet available.

COMPARISON OF LAPAROSCOPIC VERSUS OPEN APPROACH FOR SPECIFIC RESECTION TYPES

The difficulty in interpreting the meta-analyses mentioned earlier is partly because of the wide variety of procedures included. It would be useful to examine the studies comparing both approaches to the same procedure. Although issues with selection bias remain, these studies will allow a more detailed comparison.

Open Versus Laparoscopic Left Lateral Sectionectomy

As early as 2003, the group from Hopital Henri Mondor published a small case-control study examining patients undergoing anatomic resection of segments II and III through open and laparoscopic access.[13] Patients with benign lesions, HCC, and colorectal metastases were included. The findings were as follows:

1. Surgical time was longer in the laparoscopic group by approximately 1 hour ($P<.01$).
2. Perioperative blood loss was less in the laparoscopic group by approximately 200 mL ($P<.05$).
3. The length of hospital stay was not different but was relatively long in both cases (laparoscopic, 8 ± 3 days; open, 10 ± 6 days; $P =$ not significant).
4. No difference in postoperative complication rates were seen between groups.

Open Versus Laparoscopic Right Hemihepatectomy

Two recent single-center studies have compared moderate-sized series of laparoscopic and open right hemihepatectomies. The first was published in 2009 by the group from University Paris-Sud and examined 72 patients, 22 of whom underwent laparoscopic resection.[14] The patients were matched for sex, age, body mass index, American Society of Anesthesiologists score, presence of liver disease, and tumor size. In the laparoscopic group, they found similar operative times, less blood loss but a similar number of transfusions, shorter hospital stay, and a lower number of total complications with a similar number of liver specific complications (eg, decompensation, biliary leaks, bleeding).

The second study was published in 2011 and compared 36 patients undergoing laparoscopic right hemihepatectomy and 34 matched patients undergoing standard open right hemihepatectomy.[15] This study confirmed the decrease in postoperative length of stay in the laparoscopic group (5 vs 9 days; $P<.0001$). Estimated blood loss and rate of transfusion were similar between groups, and the operative times were greater in the laparoscopic group by nearly 2 hours (laparoscopic group, 300 minutes; open group, 180 minutes; $P<.0001$). The total complication rate was not different between groups.

A LOOK AT THE MOST RECENT SERIES COMPARING LAPAROSCOPIC TO OPEN HEPATECTOMY

Two recent series have compared laparoscopic and open hepatectomy. The first is from Bhojani and colleagues[16] and used a 2-to-1 matched-pair analysis to evaluate their single-center experience in Toronto. The study compared 57 laparoscopic cases, ranging from simple wedge resection to formal hemihepatectomy, with 114 open cases matched for background liver histology, number of segments resected, age, and year of procedure. The laparoscopic group had significantly less blood loss (250 vs 500 mL; $P<.001$), but no difference was seen in the rate of intraoperative transfusion or duration of the procedure. However, 24% of patients in the laparoscopic group required blood postoperatively, which was significantly more than in the open group ($P = .048$). The postoperative complication rate was similar, but the length of hospital stay was shorter in the laparoscopic group by 1 day. A cost analysis showed that laparoscopic resection also confers a cost savings if performed with parameters similar to those in the study.

A second recent study compared 27 patients who underwent laparoscopic resections versus 49 who underwent open hepatectomy. These investigators examined not only the index hospitalizations but also readmissions up to 1 year.[17] They found that the laparoscopic group had significantly less blood loss than the open group (311 vs 1086 mL; $P = .003$), and a shorter length of hospital stay (5 vs 8 days; $P = .045$). The rate of postoperative complications was similar between groups. The readmission rates at 1 year were significantly higher in the open group (39% vs 15%; $P = .02$). These readmissions were primarily for factors relating to the surgical procedure, such as drain placements, endoscopies, and incisional hernia repair. Although these issues should certainly be factored into the complex equation of decision making regarding the use of laparoscopic hepatectomy, the readmission rates and mortality rates in this series are much higher than those reported in other series, and therefore may not be generalizable (1-year readmission rate in the open group for surgery-related reasons was 53%, with a 1-year mortality rate of 10%).

PLACING LAPAROSCOPIC HEPATECTOMY FOR MALIGNANCY INTO PERSPECTIVE

A review of the worldwide literature on laparoscopic hepatectomy as conducted in 2008 found that only 45% of the total cases reported were for malignant disease.[7] Of those, approximately half were for HCC and a third for metastatic colorectal cancer, making the HCC cases only 22% of the total cases reported and colorectal metastases only 12%. The group at the University of Pittsburgh Medical Center reported that only approximately one-third of their laparoscopic resections were for malignant disease.[18]

When examined as a percentage of the total number of resections performed for cancer, the laparoscopic resections still mainly constitute a small fraction. Nguyen and colleagues[18] reported that only 25% of all patients undergoing hepatic resection at their center are believed to be candidates for a laparoscopic approach. The group from Oslo reported in 2010 that only 8% of patients with hepatic metastatic disease from colorectal cancer were undergoing laparoscopic resection, despite the group's expertise in the field.[19] Other groups have reported similarly low numbers of patients with colorectal metastatic disease who are believed to be candidates for laparoscopic hepatectomy, which have ranged from 8% to 33%.

LAPAROSCOPIC HEPATIC RESECTION FOR HCC
Concern About the Application of Laparoscopic Hepatectomy to This Subset

Because of the preponderance of abnormal hepatic parenchyma in patients with HCC, the application of laparoscopic hepatectomy to this population was not obvious. Concerns about parenchymal hemorrhage in these patients were heightened because of the presence of portal hypertension and coagulopathy. Further, trepidation existed that the pneumoperitoneum would further impair the already deranged hepatic blood flow, activate the overactivated renin-aldosterone pathway, and even potentiate the development of hepatorenal syndrome. However, open surgery in these patients is known to be deleterious and is clearly associated with hepatic decompensation, ascitic leak and subsequent infection, and renal compromise.

Results of Largest Series of Laparoscopic Hepatectomies for HCC

Despite the complexity of the concerns, several pioneering groups of hepatobiliary surgeons forged ahead and studied the application of laparoscopic techniques to hepatic resections in these difficult patients. The largest series published to date is a compilation from 3 European centers, in which laparoscopic resection was undertaken in 163 patients with HCC.[20] Of these, 74% were cirrhotic, but only those with compensated cirrhosis, moderate portal hypertension (grade I or lower varices, platelet count $\geq 80 \times 10^9$/L), and tumors less than 10 cm located away from major vascular structures were included. Anatomic liver resections were performed in 66%, and 10% had a major liver resection (≥ 3 segments). Operative blood loss was only 250 mL, and a mere 10% of patients received a transfusion. A totally laparoscopic approach was used in 95% of patients, and conversion to an open procedure was required in 9%. Length of hospital stay was 7 days and the perioperative mortality rate was 2%. Nearly 22% of patients experienced a postoperative complication, with most being low-grade (Clavien I, II, and III).

Findings of a Meta-Analysis Comparing Laparoscopic With Open Hepatectomy for HCC

As laparoscopic hepatectomy matured, it was increasingly applied to patients with HCC. Several groups began to report perioperative outcomes in small cohorts of patients. Recently, a meta-analysis reviewed the published literature until late 2010, and 9 studies comparing the outcomes of laparoscopic and open hepatectomy in patients with HCC were pooled.[21] A total of 227 patients in this analysis underwent laparoscopic hepatectomy, with 363 having open hepatectomy. The relevant findings are as follows:

1. No difference was seen in operative time between the laparoscopic and open groups.
2. Patients undergoing a laparoscopic resection had fewer positive margins than the open group (9% vs 18%; 95% CI, 0.12–0.69).
3. The laparoscopic group had significantly less blood loss (361 vs 603 mL) and required fewer transfusions (10% vs 21%; 95% CI, 0.24–0.59).
4. Patients undergoing laparoscopic hepatectomy had a shorter hospital stay and fewer overall complications (15% vs 25%; 95% CI, 0.31–0.66).
5. Most significantly, the laparoscopic group had significantly lower rates of liver failure (4% vs. 15%; 95% CI, 0.11–0.44) and postoperative ascites (5% vs 23%; 95% CI,

0.10–0.40). No difference was seen in the rates of postoperative hemorrhage and bile leak.

6. Finally, findings seemed to suggest, although they fell just short of statistical significance, that the 30-day mortality rate was lower for the laparoscopic group (OR, 0.44; 95% CI, 0.17–1.11).

Comparison of 3- and 5-Year Survivals

Although improvements in perioperative outcomes are important, long-term survival must not be compromised to achieve this. In the meta-analysis described earlier, overall and disease-free survivals at 1, 2, 3, and 5 years are described.[21] To summarize, no difference was seen in survival between the open and laparoscopic groups at any time point.

Since the publication of this meta-analysis, 2 articles have been published comparing survival after laparoscopic and open resection of HCC. The first, published by the group at University of Pittsburgh Medical Center, showed a slight disease-free survival advantage for the laparoscopic group, but no difference in overall survival at 3 years.[18] Because patients were selected based on patient and tumor factors for the laparoscopic approach, this finding should be interpreted with caution because it likely reflects selection bias. Subsequently, Lee and colleagues[22] from Hong Kong published a comparison of 33 patients who underwent laparoscopic hepatectomy for HCC and 50 patients who underwent open resection for the same indication. This study confirmed the shorter length of stay and lower postoperative morbidity observed in the meta-analysis. Further, no differences in disease-free or overall survival rates were noted at 1, 3, and 5 years.

Limitations of the Studies to Date

Although the data suggest an important role for laparoscopic hepatectomy for patients with HCC, the limitations of the data presented are important to outline. Foremost is the fact that these resections were largely performed by very experienced laparoscopic liver surgeons who pioneered the technique in the field. Second, most of the resections performed were minor resections, with only a fraction of patients undergoing a major hepatectomy. Third, patients were carefully selected for a laparoscopic approach using narrow criteria and seasoned surgical judgment. All of these factors clearly limit the generalizability of the results but suggest that in the proper clinical setting, better outcomes can potentially be achieved for certain patients with HCC through using laparoscopic techniques.

LAPAROSCOPIC HEPATIC RESECTION FOR COLORECTAL METASTASES
Concern About the Application of Laparoscopic Hepatectomy

The application of laparoscopic hepatectomy to patients with metastatic colorectal disease has been adopted more slowly and cautiously than for other indications. Because enough concern existed about the safety of laparoscopic resection of colon and rectal primary tumors to warrant a large scale randomized trial, surgeons were justifiably cautious about the application of laparoscopy to hepatic metastatic disease until the trial results were available. This area continued to be a source of controversy in the literature, with some arguing that reliable evidence, in the form of a randomized cohort or at least a prospective trial, is needed to demonstrate the safety and efficacy of laparoscopic hepatectomy in this patient subset. Proponents of the technique have countered that this type of randomized trial is not feasible because of issues such as patient preference and cost. They reason that the surgical community can extrapolate from the Clinical Outcomes of Surgical Therapy (COST) trial that there is nothing fundamentally problematic with laparoscopic resection of cancers, and further, that the safety and efficacy can be inferred from the retrospective data published to date.

Description of Large Series of Laparoscopic Hepatectomies in Patients with Metastatic Colorectal Cancer

Compared with the series for HCC, relatively few studies focusing on laparoscopic hepatectomy for patients with metastatic colorectal cancer have been reported. The largest study with the longest follow-up is from the group in Oslo.[19] They performed 117 nonanatomic and 34 anatomic liver resections (nearly all of which were left lateral sectionectomies), with a 4% conversion rate and an R0 resection rate of 93%. Sixty percent of patients had a solitary metastasis and the median size of the largest tumor was only 3 cm. Patients were followed closely for 5 years, but the median follow-up for the study as published was only 2 years. The reported 5-year recurrence rates were compared with those expected based on previously described scoring systems, and were believed to be better than expected.

A second important publication was the multi-institutional and international reports of minimally invasive liver resection in patients with metastatic colorectal cancer by Nguyen and colleagues[23] in 2009. This group performed many more major hepatic resections, with 29% having a formal right hemihepatectomy and 9% a left hemihepatectomy. Two-thirds of the patients had received preoperative chemotherapy, and 95% had previous colonic surgery. Just more than half were performed purely laparoscopically, with 40% of cases using a hand-assisted approach. Only 10% of patients received blood transfusions, and the R0 resection rate was 94%. The survival data are comparable to those seen after open hepatic resection.

Data from Studies Comparing Cohorts of Open and Laparoscopic Resections for Metastatic Colorectal Cancer

Although the outcomes presented by the large laparoscopic series just described are reasonable, comparisons between the open and laparoscopic approach are difficult to make without additional data.

The study by Castaing and colleagues[24] provides the best evidence on the safety and efficacy of laparoscopic hepatectomy in this patient population to date. They case-matched a group of 60 patients undergoing laparoscopic hepatectomy with those undergoing an open approach. Importantly, the rate of major hepatectomy was similar between groups (43% in the laparoscopic group and 38% in the open), but significantly more nonanatomic resections were performed in the laparoscopic group. In the laparoscopic group, 20% of patients underwent a simultaneous colonic resection. The severity, type, and rate of complications were nearly identical, as was the mortality rate (at 1.6%). No difference was seen in the rate of postoperative recurrence or in 5-year survival between groups. This study represents the best evidence to date that there is equivalence in the oncologic outcomes, regardless of the mode of abdominal access. Two other less mature series comparing survival after laparoscopic hepatectomy versus the open approach show similar results.[18,25]

TECHNIQUES FOR LAPAROSCOPIC HEPATECTOMY
Basic Principles

As with any new surgical procedure, the technique of laparoscopic liver resection is still evolving. It is impacted by surgical experience and the introduction of new technologies. However, the basic surgical principles that guide a laparoscopic liver resection are no different from those that guide open resection: exploration and identification of relevant tumors and their borders, mobilization of the liver, identification and transection of the hepatic vasculature inflow/outflow, parenchymal transection, and assurance of hemostasis. These goals can be accomplished through a variety of surgical approaches, including pure laparoscopic, hand-assisted laparoscopic, or laparoscopy-assisted open liver resection.

Types of Surgical Approaches

Because of the difficulties encountered in using traditional laparoscopic instruments for retracting the bulky right hemiliver, many surgeons began using hand-assisted laparoscopic approaches to help resolve some of these technical difficulties.[26] The placement of an intra-abdominal hand has several distinct advantages in the conduct of laparoscopic hepatectomy, including palpation of the tumor and assessment of margin adequacy, control of hemorrhage with compression, liver retraction that is atraumatic and dynamic, and the eventual extraction of the intact specimen. The development of lower profile and more ergonomic hand-port devices made hand-assisted laparoscopy more appealing to surgeons, and it has since been widely used by hepatic surgeons, especially those with traditional training primarily in open hepatic surgery. The use of a hand-assisted approach is thought to improve the slope of the learning curve, and may therefore make the introduction of laparoscopic hepatic resection into practice safer.[27] Pure laparoscopic approaches also have been used with increasing frequency, as experience with the procedure has increased.[28,29] Improving laparoscopic instrumentation, including robotic approaches, continues to result in iterative change to the conduct of the procedure at many experienced centers. Another technique, described as "laparoscopy-assisted" or hybrid approaches, has also been well described.[30,31] This approach uses varying amounts of laparoscopic mobilization to assist in limiting the incision size for open hepatectomy. Usually this involves an initial phase of laparoscopic mobilization of the attachments of the right hemiliver and division of the short hepatic veins, followed by open pedicle ligation and parenchymal transection through a limited open incision.

Division of Portal Pedicles

As in open hepatic surgery, several approaches to dividing the portal pedicles laparoscopically have been described. Some authors have described traditional extrahepatic dissection and ligation of the portal structures using a combination of clips, coagulation, and vascular staplers.[32,33] Others have used a similar method of extrahepatic ligation of the vascular structures, with intrahepatic ligation of the relevant biliary structures. The use of intrahepatic pedicular ligation has also been described laparoscopically, and can be used when tumors are remote from the inflow structures. A variant of this technique is to use a combination of the hand-assist device and ultrasound to help accurately locate and bloodlessly surround the pedicle of interest.[34] A precise understanding of the vascular and biliary anatomy preoperatively is essential to planning the appropriate strategy for portal pedicle ligation laparoscopically.

Technical Challenges in Laparoscopic Hepatectomy

During the development of this technique, some challenges specific to laparoscopic hepatic resection have arisen. One of the most significant is access to the posterosuperior liver segments (segments I, VII, VIII, and IVa). Because there is more limited laparoscopic visualization of these segments, lesions in these segments have been among the last to be approached laparoscopically. Some groups have described the use of lateral positioning, the use of alternative port locations (posteriorly, transpleurally), and the use of a flexible endoscope to facilitate resection of lesions in these difficult locations.[35,36] Another important challenge in purely laparoscopic liver resection is the loss of manual palpation of the liver and the relevant tumors. To help address this issue and facilitate adequate oncologic margins, a combination of detailed preoperative axial imaging and the liberal use of intraoperative ultrasound has been used by many groups. Another less pervasive challenge has been the difficulty in performing anatomic segmental resections in locations other than the segment III. Specifically, because a right hepatectomy may be more easily performed laparoscopically than a segment VI resection or a posterior sectionectomy (segments VI and VII), concern for unnecessary parenchymal resection to facilitate a minimally invasive approach has been raised.[37] Finally, the approach to occlusion of the hepatic veins has also posed a new challenge laparoscopically. Although the hepatic veins can be dissected laparoscopically, they are difficult to surround and occlude because of the loss of the ability to do this from the anterior surface. Because the traditional open view of the junction of the hepatic veins with the cava (as seen by pulling down on the liver and pushing up on the diaphragm) is more difficult to obtain laparoscopically, the hepatic veins are most easily approached posteriorly. Although these veins can also be successfully occluded from that position, it is not always possible to safely visualize their origins and occlude them without risking injury, avulsion, or incomplete ligation.

Lessons Learned to Date

Significant progress has been made recently that has allowed the introduction and adoption of techniques for laparoscopic liver resection, and in the process, some difficult lessons have been learned. Several groups have reported significant hemorrhagic complications during laparoscopic resections that were potentially more severe than would have been expected if they occurred during traditional open hepatectomy, such as large-volume hemorrhage, necessitating conversion, reoperation, and transfusion. Although in many series comparing laparoscopic and open resections the mean blood loss is less in the laparoscopic group, the upper end of the range reported in many laparoscopic series exceeds that reported in open series for cases of similar difficulty. Of the hemorrhagic events reported in the literature, the most common difficulties encountered were control of the portal veins and division of the hepatic veins, and a smaller incidence of hepatic parenchymal bleeding. Several authors have described patient deaths related to intraoperative bleeding that have occurred during the course of laparoscopic hepatic resections, and have discussed the issues relating to the learning curve, particularly as it relates to control and avoidance of intraoperative hemorrhage.

ONGOING CLINICAL TRIALS

Several clinical trials examining laparoscopic hepatic resections are currently underway. One important trial, Oslo-CoMet, is a randomized trial of open versus laparoscopic liver resection for colorectal metastases, with the primary end point of perioperative morbidity. The trial is currently accruing and is planned to enroll 340 patients in Norway, with the estimated closure date in December of 2014. A similar randomized trial comparing laparoscopic versus open hepatic resection for HCC is currently accruing and is planned to recruit nearly 200 patients in Seoul, Korea. The primary end point of this trial is recurrence at 2 years, with the targeted completion date in 2016. A final interesting ongoing clinical trial is examining the technique of laparoscopic pedicle ligation and comparing it with laparoscopic extrahepatic hilar dissection and ligation in patients with benign or malignant disease. It is being conducted in China with plans to enroll 80 patients and a target completion date of December 2017.

SUMMARY

The current literature examining the outcomes of laparoscopic hepatic resection suffers from tremendous selection bias, and in many ways the evolution of laparoscopic liver surgery is an example of how difficult the introduction of new technology can be in surgical fields. However, laparoscopic liver surgery does seem to have some advantages in selected patient groups and is likely here to stay. Currently, in experienced centers and with careful patient selection, it seems to be reasonably safe. Advantages of the laparoscopic approach seem to be reduced blood loss and shorter hospitalization. Convincing data for oncologic equivalence are currently lacking, but are likely achievable in experienced hands. Ongoing clinical trials and accumulating international experience will certainly add more definitive data. Excellence in minimally invasive liver surgery requires both significant experience with open hepatobiliary surgery and familiarity with a large variety of minimally invasive surgical techniques.

REFERENCES

1. Gagner M, Rheault M, Dubuc J. Laparoscopic partial hepatectomy for liver tumor. Surg Endosc 1992;6:99.
2. Azagra JS, Goergen M, Gilbart, et al. Laparoscopic anatomical (hepatic) left lateral segmentectomy – technical aspects. Surg Endosc 1996;10:758–61.
3. Huscher CG, Lirici MM, Chiodini S, et al. Current position of advanced laparoscopic surgery of the liver. J R Coll Surg Edinb 1997;42:219–25.
4. Cherqui D, Husson E, Hammoud R. Laparoscopic liver resections: a feasibility study in 30 patients. Ann Surg 2000;232:753–62.
5. Koffron AJ, Auffenberg G, Kung R, et al. Evaluation of 300 minimally invasive liver resections at a single institution. Ann Surg 2007;246:385–94.
6. Buell JF, Thomas MT, Rudich S, et al. Experience with more than 500 minimally invasive hepatic procedures. Ann Surg 2008;248:475–86.
7. Nguyen KT, Gamblin TC, Geller DA. World review of laparoscopic liver resection – 2,804 patients. Ann Surg 2009;250:831–41.
8. Buell JF, Cherqui D, Geller DA, et al. The international position on laparoscopic liver surgery. Ann Surg 2009;250:825–30.
9. Donadon M, Botea F, Belliappa V, et al. Experience with more than 500 minimally invasive hepatic procedures: a serious note of caution. Ann Surg 2009;249:1064–5.
10. Abdalla EK. The truth about radiofrequency ablation and laparoscopic liver resection. Ann Surg 2011;253:841–2.
11. Mirnezami R, Mirnezami AH, Chandrakumaran K, et al. Short and long-term outcomes after laparoscopic and open hepatic resection: systematic review and meta-analysis. HPB (Oxford) 2011;13:295–308.
12. Rao A, Rao G, Ahmed I, et al. Laparoscopic or open liver resection? Let systematic review decide it. Am J Surg 2012;204:222–31.
13. Lesurtel M, Cherqui D, Laurent A, et al. Laparoscopic versus open left lateral hepatic lobectomy: a case-control study. J Am Coll Surg 2003;196:236–42.
14. Dagher I, Giuro GD, Dubrez J, et al. Laparoscopic versus open right hepatectomy: a comparative study. Am J Surg 2009;198:173–7.
15. Hilal MA, Fabio FD, Teng MJ. Single-centre comparative study of laparoscopic versus open right hepatectomy. J Gastrointest Surg 2011;15:818–23.
16. Bhojani FD, Fox A, Pitzul K, et al. Clinical and economic comparison of laparoscopic to open liver resections using a 2-to-1 matched pair analysis: an institutional experience. J Am Coll Surg 2012;214:184–95.

17. Gustafson JD, Fox JP, Ouellette JP, et al. Open versus laparoscopic liver resection: looking beyond the immediate postoperative period. Surg Endosc 2012;26: 468–72.
18. Nguyen KT, Marsh JW, Tsung A, et al. Comparative benefits of laparoscopic vs open hepatic resection. Arch Surg 2011;146:348–56.
19. Kazaryan AM, Marangos IP, Rosok BI, et al. Laparoscopic resection of colorectal liver metastases. Surgical and long-term oncologic outcome. Ann Surg 2010;252: 1005–12.
20. Dagher I, Belli G, Fantini C, et al. Laparoscopic hepatectomy for hepatocellular carcinoma: a European experience. J Am Coll Surg 2010;211:16–23.
21. Fancellu A, Rosman AS, Sanna V, et al. Meta-analysis of trials comparing minimally-invasive and open liver resections for hepatocellular carcinoma. J Surg Res 2011;141:e33–45.
22. Lee KF, Chong CN, Wong J, et al. Long-term results of laparoscopic hepatectomy versus open hepatectomy for hepatocellular carcinoma: a case-match analysis. World J Surg 2011;35:2268–74.
23. Nguyen KT, Laurent A, Dagher I, et al. Minimally invasive liver resection for metastatic colorectal cancer. A multi-institutional, international report of safety, feasibility and early outcomes. Ann Surg 2009;250:842–8.
24. Castaing D, Vibert E, Ricca L, et al. Oncologic results of laparoscopic versus open hepatectomy for colorectal liver metastases in two specialized centers. Ann Surg 2009;250:849–55.
25. Huh JW, Koh YS, Kim HR, et al. Comparison of laparoscopic and open colorectal resections for patients undergoing simultaneous R0 resection for liver metastases. Surg Endosc 2011;25:193–8.
26. Fong Y, Jarnagin W, Blumgart L. Hand-assisted laparoscopic liver surgery. Operat Tech Gen Surg 2002;4(1):88–98.
27. Buell JF, Koffron AJ, Thomas MJ, et al. Laparoscopic liver resection. J Am Coll Surg 2005;200:472–80.
28. Gayet B, Cavaliere D, Vibert E, et al. How I do it: totally laparoscopic right hepatectomy. Am J Surg 2007;194:685–9.
29. Dagher I, Caillard C, Proske J, et al. Laparoscopic right hepatectomy: original technique and results. J Am Coll Surg 2008;206:756–60.
30. Koffron AJ, Kung RD, Auffenberg GB. Laparoscopic liver surgery for everyone: the hybrid method. Surgery 2007;142:463–8.
31. Nitta H, Sasaki A, Fujita T, et al. Laparoscopy-assisted major liver resections employing a hanging technique. The original procedure. Ann Surg 2010;251: 450–3.
32. O'Rourke N, Fielding G. Laparoscopic right hepatectomy: surgical technique. J Gastrointest Surg 2004;8:213–6.
33. Pearce NW, Fabio FD, Hilal MA. Laparoscopic left hepatectomy with extraparenchymal inflow control. J Am Coll Surg 2011;213:e23–27.
34. Belli G, Limongelli P, Fantini C, et al. Laparoscopic and open treatment of hepatocellular carcinoma in patients with cirrhosis. Br J Surg 2009;96:1041–8.
35. Kazaryan AM, Rosok BI, Marangos IP, et al. Comparative evaluation of laparoscopic liver resection for posterosuperior and anterolateral segments. Surg Endosc 2011;25:3881–9.
36. Cho JY, Han HS, Yoon YS, et al. Feasibility of laparoscopic liver resection for tumors located in the posterosuperior segments of the liver, with a special reference to overcoming current limitations on tumor location. Surgery 2008;144: 32–8.

37. Zalinski S, Mariette C, Farges O, et al. Management of patients with synchronous liver metastases of colorectal cancer. Clinical practice guidelines. Guidelines of the French society of gastrointestinal surgery (SFCD) and of the association of hepatobiliary surgery and liver transplantation (ACHBT). Short version. J Visc Surg 2011;148:e171–182.

Technique, Outcomes, and Evolving Role of Extirpative Laparoscopic and Robotic Surgery for Renal Cell Carcinoma

Youssef S. Tanagho, MD, MPH, R. Sherburne Figenshau, MD,
Sam B. Bhayani, MD*

KEYWORDS

- Extirpative laparoscopic surgery • Robotic surgery • Renal carcinoma
- Radical nephrectomy • Partial nephrectomy

KEY POINTS

- Laparoscopic renal surgery is associated with decreased blood loss, shorter hospital stay, improved cosmesis, and more rapid convalescence relative to open renal surgery.
- Laparoscopic partial nephrectomy is a minimally invasive, nephron-sparing alternative to laparoscopic radical nephrectomy for the treatment of small renal masses.
- While offering similar oncologic outcomes to laparoscopic radical nephrectomy, the technical challenges and steep learning curve associated with laparoscopic partial nephrectomy limits its wider dissemination.
- Robot-assisted partial nephrectomy, although still an evolving procedure with no long-term data, has emerged as a viable alternative to laparoscopic partial nephrectomy, with favorable initial outcomes.

INTRODUCTION

Because of the increased detection of small renal masses on abdominal imaging, the incidence of renal cell carcinoma has increased significantly in recent years. Accompanying this trend is a clear stage migration favoring stage I tumors and a significant decrease in tumor size even within the stage I group.[1] By 2007, 13.5% of newly diagnosed renal tumors measured less than 2 cm, 37% less than 3 cm, and close to 60% less than 4 cm.[2]

Disclosures: Funding sources: Conflict of Interest: Dr Tanagho: None: Dr Tanagho: None: Dr Figenshau: None: Dr Figenshau: None Dr Bhayani: None Dr Bhayani: None.
Division of Urologic Surgery, Washington University School of Medicine, 660 South Euclid Avenue, St Louis, MO 63110, USA
* Corresponding author.
E-mail address: bhayani@wustl.edu

Surg Oncol Clin N Am 22 (2013) 91–109
http://dx.doi.org/10.1016/j.soc.2012.08.002
1055-3207/13/$ – see front matter © 2013 Elsevier Inc. All rights reserved.

The gold standard for the treatment of renal tumors traditionally has been radical nephrectomy. Investigation over the last decade, however, has found the surgical feasibility and equivalent oncologic efficacy of partial nephrectomy for small renal masses.[3] Furthermore, a growing body of evidence has suggested that overtreatment of renal masses with radical nephrectomy is associated with increased risk of chronic renal insufficiency, cardiovascular events, and premature deaths.[4–6] Accordingly, the American Urological Association guidelines now explicitly place partial nephrectomy as the standard of care for managing T1a renal tumors (<4 cm) and as an alternative treatment option for T1b tumors (4–7 cm).[7] Reflecting this paradigm shift, the use of partial nephrectomy has increased substantially at many centers of excellence over the last decade, approaching 90% for T1a tumors at some centers.[8] Nevertheless, radical nephrectomy remains the standard of care for managing tumors greater than 7 cm in size, tumors extending into the renal vein, and tumors invading Gerota's fascia or adjacent organs.[7]

In 1990, Clayman and colleagues[9] performed the first laparoscopic radical nephrectomy (LRN), showing the feasibility of this minimally invasive alternative to open radical nephrectomy (ORN). With the rapid uptake of minimally invasive technology by the urologic community, laparoscopic partial nephrectomy (LPN), first reported in 1993,[10] and robot-assisted partial nephrectomy (RAPN), first performed in 2004,[11] emerged as viable alternatives to open partial nephrectomy (OPN) for the management of suspected renal malignancy. The long-term oncologic and functional outcomes of minimally invasive renal surgery are comparable with those of open renal surgery,[12,13] with the potential benefits of estimated blood loss (EBL), shorter hospital stay (LOS), improved cosmesis, and more rapid convalescence. Herein, we review the technique and outcomes of LRN, LPN, and RAPN, evaluating the current role and future prospects of each of these approaches for the treatment of renal malignancy.

LAPAROSCOPIC RADICAL NEPHRECTOMY
Principles in Surgical Technique

LRN can be performed for most patients with organ-confined T1–T3a renal tumors who are not candidates for nephron-sparing surgery.[14] Previously considered contraindications to LRN, larger organ-confined tumors and tumors with renal vein thrombus may be amenable to a laparoscopic approach, depending on individual surgeon experience.[15]

Preoperative assessment of pulmonary and cardiac function before LRN (and minimally invasive renal surgery in general) is essential, as the pneumoperitoneum, combined with the lateral decubitus position characteristic of minimally invasive renal surgery, can impact patients with severe cardiopulmonary disease by compromising ventilation and venous return. Patients with chronic pulmonary disease may be unable to compensate for pneumoperitoneum-induced hypercarbia and may require lowering of pneumoperitoneum pressures, use of helium as an insufflant, or open conversion.[16,17]

A transperitoneal or retroperitoneal approach is chosen depending on tumor location, patient surgical history, and surgeon preference. Although safe and effective in experienced hands, the retroperitoneal approach is potentially more challenging because of its confined workspace and relatively fewer anatomic landmarks.[18] The transperitoneal approach is the most widely used approach for minimally invasive renal surgery.

The most commonly used camera and trocar configuration for the transperitoneal approach places the camera in a medial position, superior to the umbilicus; a 30°

downward-angled lens is used. Two additional trocars are placed just cephalad of the anterior superior iliac spine and a few centimeters below the costal margin in the mid-axillary line. During transperitoneal LRN, the peritoneum is incised sharply along the line of Toldt and the bowel mobilized medially, thus developing the avascular plane between Gerota's fascia and the posterior mesocolon. For right-sided tumors, mobilization of the duodenum may be necessary. Attachments between the renal upper pole and the liver/spleen are then released. Further medial reflection of the mesentery exposes the ureter and gonadal vein. The ureter is lifted, exposing the psoas muscle, and the dissection is continued proximally toward the renal hilum. The renal vein can be identified by tracing the gonadal vein cranially to its insertion in the renal vein on the left side and the inferior vena cava, in proximity to the right renal vein, on the right side. With the kidney on stretch, the renal vein and more posteriorly located renal artery are dissected. The renal artery and, subsequently, renal vein are clipped and transected. Importantly, large hilar tumors distorting the renal hilum must be approached cautiously to avoid transection of aberrant major aortic branches. The ureter is then clipped and transected.[19]

For retroperitoneal LRN, access is obtained through a 1.2-cm skin incision just below the tip of the 12th rib. The flank muscle fibers and thoracolumbar fascia are bluntly split, and the surgeon's fingertip creates a potential space between the psoas muscle and Gerota's fascia; this space is further developed by injection of 800 mL of air into the retroperitoneum through a balloon dilator. The camera port is then placed at the site of the balloon dilator. Two additional working ports are triangulated with the camera at an obtuse angle to minimize clashing of the instruments. When performing retroperitoneal LRN, the renal hilum is approached posteriorly after development of a working space between Gerota's fascia and the psoas muscle and subsequent exposure of the ureter and gonadal vein. In contrast to the transperitoneal approach, the renal artery is usually encountered before the renal vein during retroperitoneal LRN given the posterior relationship of the artery to the vein.[20,21]

Established guidelines for renal cancer surgery, including preservation of tumor integrity and Gerota's fascia, must be applied to achieve the best oncologic outcomes. To avoid contact with the abdominal wall, the excised surgical specimen must be removed in an impermeable sac.[22,23] Either intact specimen extraction or specimen morcellation may be performed safely,[24] although extreme caution must be exercised to avoid sac perforation with potential tumor spillage if morcellation is to be performed.[15]

Oncologic Outcomes

The oncologic efficacy of LRN seems to be equivalent to that of the traditional ORN. In a multicenter study comparing the oncologic outcomes of 64 patients who underwent LRN with 69 patients who underwent ORN, Portis and colleagues[25] reported a Kaplan-Meier–estimated 5-year disease-free survival of 92% and 91%, respectively; respective cancer specific survival was 98% versus 92%. The authors concluded that LRN does not increase the risk of local tumor recurrence or distant metastasis.

LRN does not seem to result in a significant risk of port-site seeding. In a comprehensive review of port-site metastasis in urologic surgery, Tsivian and Sidi found only 3 documented cases of port-site metastasis following LRN for renal cell carcinoma.[22] The authors note that 2 of those cases occurred in patients who had undergone specimen morcellation before extraction, although the role of morcellation in contributing to these rare cases of port-site recurrences is debatable.[26,27] Others have reported that specimen morcellation does not confer an increased risk for port-site seeding when proper surgical technique is adhered to.[24]

Functional Outcomes

Comparing the renal functional outcomes of LRN and OPN for tumors measuring ≤4 cm, Matin and colleagues[28] noted that patients who underwent nephron-sparing surgery experienced less postoperative deterioration in renal function, as determined by the percentage of increase in serum creatinine level postoperatively (0% in the OPN group vs 25% in the LRN group, $P<.001$).

Regardless of surgical technique (ie, minimally invasive vs open), radical nephrectomy is clearly associated with inferior renal functional outcomes relative to partial nephrectomy. A Memorial Sloan Kettering study examining 3-year renal functional outcomes in patients undergoing radical nephrectomy versus those undergoing partial nephrectomy found a 65% probability of the development of new-onset stage 3 or higher chronic kidney disease[29] in the radical nephrectomy group compared with a 20% probability in the partial nephrectomy group ($P<.0001$).[30]

Perioperative Outcomes

LRN is clearly associated with decreased EBL, decreased LOS, and more rapid convalescence relative to ORN. A comparative perioperative assessment of 33 patients with T2 tumors (≥7 cm) who underwent LRN at the Cleveland Clinic and 34 patients who underwent ORN for tumors of similar stage at the same institution found a mean EBL of 294 mL in the laparoscopic group, compared with 837 mL in the open group; mean LOS was 1.8 days in the LRN group versus 6.1 days in the ORN cohort.[31]

A more recent comparison of 65 patients with T2 renal tumors who underwent LRN and 34 patients with tumors of equivalent stage who underwent ORN found decreased analgesic requirements ($P<.001$) and more rapid convalescence ($P = .02$) in the LRN group.[32]

Complications

Reported complication rates can vary substantially depending on prospective versus retrospective reporting and the appropriate use of standardized classification criteria.[33] Nevertheless, LRN is generally associated with a low incidence of complications when performed by surgeons experienced in minimally invasive techniques.[15] Siqueira and colleagues[34] reported a major complication rate of 4% in their review of 61 LRN cases; these included one vascular complication, one hemorrhagic complication, one visceral injury (liver injury during port placement), and one bowel injury. Steinberg and colleagues[31] reported a complication rate of 6.2% in 33 patient undergoing LRN for T2 tumors versus a complication rate of 23.5% in 34 patients undergoing ORN for tumors of equivalent stage, although the difference was not statistically significant.

LAPAROSCOPIC PARTIAL NEPHRECTOMY
Principles in Surgical Technique

Patient positioning, port placement, and kidney exposure during LPN follow the same principles as those for LRN. In contrast to LRN, Gerota's fascial must be incised and the perirenal fat swept away from the kidney during LPN to gain full exposure of the renal tumor. Care must be taken to preserve the fat directly overlying the renal lesion in anticipation of extracapsular tumor extension. With the tumor exposed, the precise position and borders of the tumor are delineated, often under intraoperative ultrasound guidance.

Traditionally, renal hilar vessels are clamped before tumor excision during partial nephrectomy. In contrast to OPN, which often is performed under conditions of renal hypothermia to minimize ischemic insult to the clamped kidney, minimally invasive techniques for achieving renal hypothermia during renal hilar clamping have failed to achieve widespread clinical application.

In recognition of the potential impact that even a limited duration of warm ischemia time may have on renal function,[35,36] variations in surgical technique have been attempted to minimize or eliminate warm ischemia during LPN. Some investigators have adopted an early unclamping technique, whereby the hilar vessels are only clamped during sharp dissection of the tumor from kidney and while suturing obvious vessels and the collecting system at the resection base. Gill and colleagues[37] were able to decrease their warm ischemia time for LPN from 31.6 to 14.4 minutes using this technique. Others have described successful use of a selective renal parenchymal clamping technique, whereby the renal parenchyma is regionally clamped only in the area of the planned excision. Benway and colleagues[38] reported improved renal functional outcomes with segmental rather than complete hilar clamping in a porcine model, whereas Figenshau showed the safety and feasibility of this technique in humans.[39] More recently, some surgeons have performed LPN without any clamping of the renal hilum, often in the setting of medically induced hypotension, and have suggested that off-clamp, zero-ischemia, LPN can be safely performed in carefully selected patients.[40] Nevertheless, multiple studies in humans have failed to demonstrate long-term improvement in renal functional outcomes after any modification of clamping technique or in the absence of renal hilar clamping.[35,41,42] Additional studies are needed to establish the efficacy and reaffirm the safety of these unconventional and, arguably, still experimental surgical approaches.

Traditionally, 12.5 g of mannitol is administered intravenously 15–20 minutes before renal hilar clamping, because this is believed to minimize reperfusion injury after release of the renal vascular clamps. Tumor excision is performed sharply with a rim of normal renal parenchyma, with simultaneous use of electrocautery to facilitate hemostasis. Hemostatic agents, such as gelatin matrix thrombin sealant (Floseal, Baxter; Deerfield, IL), may aid in achieving hemostasis, although larger vessels at the resection base may necessitate sutured vascular repair.

After tumor excision, renorrhaphy is traditionally performed in 2 layers. A deep-layer closure of the resection bed, including repair of large blood vessels or any collecting system defects, is first performed, followed by an outer layer closure of the renal capsule. To enhance the tension of the parenchymal closure, surgical bolsters are generally placed in the renal defect after the deep layer closure and before the outer layer closure.[19] Knotless renorrhaphy using Weck Hem-O-Lock clips (Weck Closure Systems, Research Triangle Park, NC, USA) to anchor the capsular sutures on opposite sides of the renal defect has been adopted by some to expedite the closure and, thus, reduce warm ischemia time.[43] Importantly, absorbable suture must be used during renal reconstruction, because nonabsorbable suture may serve as a nidus for stone formation.

LPN remains technically challenging, requiring considerable technical expertise to achieve adequate tumor resection, pelvicaliceal reconstruction, and parenchymal renorrhaphy while maintaining hemostasis and minimizing ischemia times during hilar clamping. Despite the development of novel techniques to facilitate LPN by expert laparoscopic surgeons, the steep learning curve associated with this technique has impeded its wider dissemination into general practices in the United States and may contribute to the underutilization of partial nephrectomy.[44]

Given its technical challenges, LPN traditionally has been performed in select patients with small, exophytic, easily accessible tumors,[45] although successful and safe application of this technique has been described for larger, more complex tumors by expert minimally invasive surgeons.[46]

Oncologic Outcomes

In a study by Gill and colleagues[47] comparing 100 early cases of LPN (median tumor size 2.8 cm) with 100 cases of OPN (median tumor size 3.3 cm), positive parenchymal margin occurred in 2 cases of LPN versus zero cases of OPN; of note, no patients in the LPN group had local tumor recurrence.

More recently, Gill and colleagues[12] compared the 3-year oncologic outcomes of 514 patients who underwent LPN and 676 patients who underwent OPN and had a Kaplan-Meier-estimated 3-year cancer specific survival of 99.3% and 99.2%, respectively. Kaplan-Meier-estimates of local recurrence were 1.4% versus 1.5%, whereas estimates of distant recurrence were 0.9% versus 2.1%, respectively.

Long-term oncologic outcomes from the largest series of LPN were recently reported by Lane and colleagues and were comparable with those of OPN. At 7-year follow-up, metastasis-free survival was 97.5% in the LPN group versus 97.3% in the OPN group ($P = .47$). Using propensity score matching to account for baseline differences between the 2 cohorts, 7-year metastasis-free survival was similar after LPN and OPN. On multivariate analysis, surgical approach (LPN vs OPN) failed to predict all-cause morality.[13]

Functional Outcomes

Comparing a cohort of 100 patients who underwent LPN with a cohort of 100 patients who underwent OPN—each with similar preoperative serum creatinine levels (1.0 vs 1.0 mg/dL, $P = .52$)—Gill and colleagues[47] reported no difference in postoperative serum creatinine level between the 2 groups (1.1 vs 1.2 mg/dL, $P = .65$).

In a more recent multicenter comparison of 771 patients who underwent LPN and 1028 patients who underwent OPN, Gill and colleagues[12] reported similar renal functional outcomes 3 months postoperatively for the patient cohort. In the LPN group, mean preoperative serum creatinine level was 1.01 compared with 1.18 postoperatively; in the OPN group, mean preoperative serum creatinine level was 1.25, compared with 1.42 postoperatively. Of note, in the subset of patients with a solitary kidney, a statistically significant advantage in renal preservation favored the OPN approach over the LPN approach. Patients with a solitary kidney who underwent LPN had a mean preoperative serum creatinine value of 1.24 versus 1.90 postoperatively, whereas those who underwent OPN had a mean preoperative creatinine value of 1.32 compared with 1.73 postoperatively. These results raise concerns about the appropriateness of the LPN approach in patients with a solitary kidney or compromised baseline renal function.

Perioperative Outcomes

In a study of 50 LPNs performed for tumors with a mean size of 3 cm, investigators reported a mean warm ischemia time of 23 minutes, a mean operating time of 3 hours, and a mean LOS of 2.2 days.[48] In the study by Gill and colleagues,[47] comparing 100 cases of LPN with 100 cases of OPN, mean operating time was 3 hours versus 3.9 hours, respectively; mean warm ischemia time was 28 versus 18 minutes; mean EBL was 125 mL versus 250 mL; mean LOS was 2 days versus 5 days; mean analgesic requirement was 20.2 mg morphine sulfate equivalent versus 252.5 mg; average convalescence was 4 weeks versus 6 weeks. This study found a clear advantage in postoperative recovery favoring the LPN approach over the OPN approach.

Similar findings were reported in the more recent analysis by Gill and colleagues[12] of 771 patients who underwent LPN and 1028 patients who underwent OPN. In this study, a mean operating time of 3.3 hours was noted in the LPN group compared with 4.3 hours in the OPN group. Mean warm ischemia time was 30.7 and 20.1 minutes in the 2 groups, respectively. Mean EBL was 300 mL in the LPN group versus 376 mL in the open group. Mean LOS was 3.3 days and 5.8 days, respectively.

Complications

An international literature review of 97 patients undergoing LPN found a major complication rate of 10%.[48] In a multicenter European study of 53 patients undergoing LPN, intraoperative bleeding was reported in 8% of patients; postoperative bleeding was noted in 2% of patients, whereas postoperative urinoma was reported in 10% of patients. Conversion to open surgery was required in 4% of patients secondary to bleeding and in 4% secondary to technical problems. Reintervention via percutaneous nephrostomy drainage occurred in 4% of patients, 2% of patients required postoperative stent placement, 4% required open revision, and 2% required nephrectomy.[49]

In their comparative study of 100 LPN cases and 100 OPN cases, Gill and colleagues[47] reported no difference in the overall incidence of postoperative complications between the 2 groups (16% vs 13%, $P = .55$). However, compared with the OPN group, the LPN cohort had a higher incidence of intraoperative complications (5% vs 0%; $P = .02$) as well as urologic postoperative complications (11% vs 2%; $P = .01$).

In their more recent comparison of 771 patients who underwent LPN and 1028 patients who underwent OPN, Gill and colleagues[12] reported an intraoperative complication rate of 1.8% in the LPN group versus 1.0% in the OPN group; the postoperative complication rate was 18.6% in the LPN group and 13.7% in the OPN group. On multivariate analysis, the odds of a postoperative complication after LPN were 1.66 (95% confidence interval [CI], 1.33–2.05) times higher than those after OPN. The odds of urologic complications were 2.14 (95% CI, 1.39–3.31) higher for LPN than for OPN, whereas the odds of nonurologic complications were 1.53 (95% CI, 1.12–2.10) higher in the LPN group. A postoperative hemorrhage rate of 4.2% was noted in the LPN group compared with 1.6% in the OPN group. On multivariate analysis, the odds of postoperative hemorrhage after LPN were 3.53 (95% CI, 1.88–4.94) times higher than for OPN. The blood transfusion rate was 5.8% in the LPN group versus 3.4% in the OPN group. Postoperative urine leakage occurred in 3.1% of patients in the LPN group compared with 2.3% in the OPN group. The odds of requiring a secondary procedure for any reason were 3.05 (95% CI, 1.88, 4.94) times higher in the LPN group than in the OPN group. Based on these cumulative results, this large multicenter study shows that LPN is, in fact, associated with increased risk of complications relative to OPN, even in expert hands.

ROBOT-ASSISTED PARTIAL NEPHRECTOMY
Principles in Surgical Technique

RAPN is performed using the da Vinci surgical system (Intuitive Surgical Inc, Sunnyvale, CA). Among its potential advantages, robotic technology offers high-definition, 3-dimensional visualization, a wider range of wristed-instrument motion, and scaling of surgeon movements. Newer robotic systems also include a fourth robotic arm (in addition to the camera arm and 2 standard working arms), which provides the surgeon an additional working channel. Nevertheless, the robotic surgeon must rely on a bedside assistant to facilitate the surgery by using conventional laparoscopic instruments to provide countertraction and suction through an additional assistant port.

As with LRN and LPN, in RAPN, a camera port is placed medial and superior to the umbilicus, and 2 trocars for the robotic arms are placed just cephalad of the anterior superior iliac spine and below the costal margin along the midaxillary line. Unique to RAPN, an additional 12-mm assistant port is placed in the midline, usually inferior to the umbilicus, although the surgeon may elect to place the assistant port in the upper quadrant depending on tumor location. If a fourth robotic arm is to be used, the trocar is placed laterally, triangulated between the 2 other robotic trocars.[19,50] The robot is then docked posterior to the patient.

The technique for RAPN, although similar to that of LPN, continues to evolve. Our current approach uses the newly developed robot-controlled ultrasound probe (Aloka, Tokyo, Japan), which allows complete surgeon control of intraoperative imaging, thereby facilitating tumor identification and delineation of the resection site. Newer robotic platforms also include TilePro software integration (Intuitive Surgical Inc, Sunnyvale, CA, USA), which allows for real-time picture-on-picture display of radiographic images on the console screen, further facilitating the mapping out of the dissection. The recent introduction of robotic Bulldog clamps may provide the surgeon additional autonomy, in lieu of having to relegate the sensitive task of hilar occlusion to the bedside assistant.

Sliding-clip renorrhaphy has been described recently as a preferable alternative to the traditional tied-suture for closure of the renal defect during RAPN. This renorrhaphy method relies on the use of Weck Hem-o-Lok clips (Weck Closure Systems, Research Triangle Park, NC, USA), placed on either side of the defect and then slid into place by the surgeon to exert tension on the repair. The Hem-o-Lok clips are generally reinforced with LapraTy clips (Ethicon; Cincinnati, OH) to prevent backsliding of the clips. Although the use of Weck Hem-o-Lok clips to facilitate renorrhaphy has been applied to LPN, the sliding-clip technique described for RAPN differs from earlier laparoscopic applications in that the surgeon controls the tension of the closure by sliding the clips into the desired position, effectively eliminating the need for placement of surgical bolsters in the renal defect to achieve tight closure. This technique is ideally suited for RAPN, as the robotic instrumentation affords the surgeon the requisite precision in dictating the degree of tension placed on the repair.[51,52] By simplifying the closure, while minimizing reliance on the assistant, sliding-clip renorrhaphy has been found to substantially reduce warm ischemia time compared with tied-suture renorrhaphy.[52] A recently described variation of the sliding-clip technique is the use of barbed suture (V-loc, Covidien; Mansfield, MA) to facilitate efficient and tight renorrhaphy without slippage of sutures or clips.[53,54]

RAPN seems to have a shorter learning curve than LPN[55] and, as such, may facilitate and promote the use of minimally invasive nephron-sparing surgery. Numerous reports describe the intraoperative and perioperative outcomes of RAPN, compare the experiences of RAPN with those of LPN, and describe the utility of RAPN in the management of complex renal masses. Nevertheless, for the inexperienced robotic renal surgeon, careful patient selection is essential. The absence of haptic feedback and reliance on the bedside assistant can present challenges unique to RAPN. Candidates ideally suited for initial RAPN procedures include patients with predominantly nonhilar, exophytic T1a lesions, uncomplicated vascular anatomy, and a normal contralateral kidney.

Oncologic Outcomes

Because RAPN is a newer technique, positive surgical margin rates have often been reported as surrogates for oncologic control. Reported positive surgical margin rates for RAPN have typically ranged from 1.2% to 5.7%.[56–59] A review of contemporary RAPN series by Benway and Bhayani[60] found that the comprehensive surgical margin rate across all studies reviewed was 2.7%. These rates are comparable with those reported by Gill and colleagues[12] for LPN and OPN—2.9% and 1.3%, respectively. Positive margin rates in various RAPN series are depicted in **Table 1**,[11,55,57,58,61–72] and studies comparing positive margin rates between RAPN and LPN are depicted in **Table 2**.[59,73–79]

Despite the use of positive surgical margin rates as a metric for assessing oncologic success, the impact of positive surgical margins on the outcomes of patients undergoing partial nephrectomy for renal cell carcinoma seems to be negligible.[80,81] Evaluating a series of more than 770 patients undergoing partial nephrectomy, Kwon and colleagues[80] observed no difference in the incidence of recurrent disease between those with positive surgical margins and those with negative margins; less aggressive tumors, in particular, were unlikely to recur irrespective of margin status. A more recent analysis suggests that recurrences after positive surgical margins are rare.[81]

Early and intermediate outcomes of RAPN show excellent oncologic control. Across more than 1600 patients detailed in the review by Benway and Bhayani[60] of modern large series, only 7 recurrences have been reported to date, a rate of less than 1%. Although these initial data are certainly encouraging, long-term data on RAPN are lacking. Long-term oncologic outcomes from the largest series of LPN were recently reported and were comparable with those of OPN.[13] Several recent studies have found that RAPN provides oncologic outcomes equivalent to LPN in the short and intermediate term.[58,64,67,69,74,76] Although it is projected that RAPN will offer similar long-term oncologic benefit as LPN, these long-term data are required for RAPN before it can be fully endorsed.

Functional Outcomes

In addition to serving as a proxy for the ease with which a surgeon is able to perform renorrhaphy during minimally invasive partial nephrectomy, warm ischemia time is a crucial metric of functional outcomes after partial nephrectomy, because longer warm ischemia times have been associated with short- and long-term renal functional decline.[35,36] The fact that OPN is often performed under conditions of renal hypothermia, while few published LPN and RAPN series use renal-cooling techniques, gives further impetus for minimally invasive renal surgeons to demonstrate acceptable warm ischemia times. A review of LPN and OPN case series found that the mean warm ischemia time for LPN was 27–35 minutes—considerably longer than the ischemia times reported for OPN.[82] Initial investigation suggests that RAPN may not require as long a learning curve as LPN to achieve a reasonable warm ischemia time.[55]

Earlier studies by Caruso and colleagues[73] and Deane and colleagues[75], which compared approximately 20 patients who underwent either RAPN or LPN, found no significant differences in warm ischemia time between the 2 groups. Similarly, Aron and colleagues[74] performed a matched cohort study of 24 patients who underwent either RAPN or LPN and found no significant differences in warm ischemia time between the 2 cohorts. A retrospective matched cohort study of 150 patients undergoing RAPN or LPN by Haber and colleagues[78] found that despite a slight advantage in warm ischemia time favoring the RAPN group (18.2 vs 20.3 minutes), the difference was not statistically significant ($P = .27$).

In contrast to the aforementioned studies, a study by Benway and colleagues[59] comparing 129 patients and 118 patients who underwent RAPN and LPN, respectively, found that mean warm ischemia time was significantly shorter in the RAPN group (19.7 vs 28.4 minutes, $P < .001$); RAPN maintained a consistently shorter mean warm ischemia time than LPN in patients with complex renal masses (25.9 vs 36.7 minutes, $P < .001$). Other smaller comparative series of RAPN and LPN have also found an advantage in warm ischemia time favoring RAPN. In a series of 40

Table 1
Contemporary robotic partial nephrectomy case series

Reference	No. of Cases	Mean Tumor Size, cm	Mean Operating Time, min	Mean WIT, min	Mean EBL, mL	Mean LOS, d	PSM, n (%)	Complications, n (%)	Mean F/U, mo
Gettman et al,[11] 2004	13	NR	215	22	170	4.3	1 (7.7)	NR	NR
Phillips et al,[61] 2005	12	1.8	265	26	240	2.7	NR	1 (8.3)	NR
Kaul et al,[62] 2007	10	2	155	21	92	1.5	0 (0)	2 (20)	15
Bhayani and Das,[63] 2008	35	2.8	142	21.0	133	2.5	None	6 (17)	NR
Rogers et al,[64] 2008	148	2.8	197	27.7	183	1.9	6 (4)	9 (6)	18
Ho et al,[65] 2009	20	3.5	82.8	21.7	189	4.8	None	None	>12
Michli and Para,[66] 2009	20	2.7	142	28	263	2.8	0 (0)	2 (10)	NR
Gong et al,[67] 2010	29	3.0	197	25.0	220	2.5	None	None	15

Study	No. of patients	Tumor size (cm)	OR time (min), median	WIT (min)	EBL (mL), median	LOS (d), median	PSM, n (%)	Complications, n (%)	F/U (mo)
Mottrie et al,[55] 2010	62	2.8	90	20	95	5	2 (3.2)	10 (16.1)	NR
Benway et al,[68] 2010	183	2.9	210	23.9	132	NR	7 (3.8)	18 (9.8)	≤26
Scoll et al,[57] 2010	100	2.8	206	25.5	127	3.2	5 (5.7)	13 (13)	12.7
Patel et al,[69] 2010	71	2.1–5	238–275	20–25	100	2	3 (4.2)	9 (12.6)	12
Petros et al,[70] 2010	95	2.3–2.5	246–250	16–21	100–150	2	NR	22 (23)	NR
Lorenzo et al,[71] 2011	65	NR	171	NR	243.2	4.6	6 (9.2)	1 (1.5)	13
Naeem et al,[72] 2011	97	2.3–2.5	243–265	22.5–26.5	100–150	2	2 (2)	8 (8.2)	12
Dulabon et al,[58] 2011 (nonhilar vs hilar)	405 vs 41	2.9 vs 3.5	187.4 vs 194.5	19.6 vs 26.3	208.2 vs 262.2	2.9 vs 2.9	6 (1.5) vs 1 (2.4)	22 (5.4) vs 1 (2.4)	≤45

Abbreviations: EBL, Estimated Blood Loss; F/U, follow-up; NR, Not Reported; PSM, Positive Surgical Margin; WIT, Warm Ischemia Time.

Table 2
Series comparing RAPN (A) Versus LPN (B)

Reference	No. of Cases	Mean Tumor Size, cm	Mean Operating Time, min	Mean WIT, min	Mean EBL, mL	Mean LOS, d	PSM, n (%)	Complications, n (%)	Mean F/U, mo
Caruso et al,[73] 2006	A: 10 B: 10	A: 2.0 B: 2.2	A: 279 B: 253	A: 26.4 B: 29.3	A: 240 B: 200	A: 2.6 B: 2.7	A: 0 (0) B: 1 (10)	A: 1 (10) B: 1 (10)	A: NR B: NR
Aron et al,[74] 2008	A: 12 B: 12	A: 2.4 B: 2.9	A: 242 B: 256	A: 23 B: 22	A: 329 B: 300	A: 4.7 B: 4.4	A: NR B: NR	A: NR B: NR	A: 7.4 B: 8.5
Deane et al,[75] 2008	A: 11 B: 11	A: 3.1 B: 2.3	A: 229 B: 290	A: 32.1 B: 35.3	A: 115 B: 198	A: 2.0 B: 3.1	A: 0 (0) B: 1 (9.1)	A: 1 (9.1) B: 1 (9.1)	A: 16 B: 4.5
Benway et al,[59] 2009	A: 129 B: 118	A: 2.9 B: 2.6	A: 189 B: 174	A: 19.7 B: 28.4	A: 155 B: 196	A: 2.4 B: 2.7	A: 5 (3.9) B: 1 (0.8)	A: 11 (8.5) B: 12 (10.2)	A: NR B: NR
Kural et al,[76] 2009	A: 11 B: 20	A: 3.2 B: 3.1	A: 185 B: 226	A: 27.3 B: 35.8	A: 286 B: 388	A: 3.9 B: 4.3	A: 0 (0) B: 1 (5)	A: 1 (9.1) B: 0 (0)	A: 7.5 B: 38
Wang and Bhayani,[77] 2009	A: 40 B: 62	A: 2.5 B: 2.4	A: 140 B: 156	A: 19 B: 25	A: 137 B: 173	A: 2.5 B: 2.9	A: 1 (2.5) B: 1 (1.6)	A: 8 (20) B: 9 (14.5)	A: NR B: NR
Haber et al,[78] 2010	A: 75 B: 75	A: 2.8 B: 2.5	A: 200 B: 197	A: 18.2 B: 20.3	A: 323 B: 222	A: 4.2 B: 4.1	A: 0 (0) B: 0 (0)	A: 12 (16.0) B: 10 (13.3)	A: NR B: NR
Williams et al,[79] 2011	A: 27 B: 59	A: 2.5 B: 3.1	A: 233 B: 221	A: 18.5 B: 28.0	A: 180 B: 146	A: 2.5 B: 2.7	A: 1 (3.7) B: 7 (11.9)	A: 5 (18.5) B: 12 (20.3)	A: NR B: NR

Abbreviations: EBL, Estimated Blood Loss; F/U, follow-up; NR, Not Reported; PSM, Positive Surgical Margin; WIT, Warm Ischemia Time.

RAPNs and 62 LPNs, Wang and Bhayani[77] reported a warm ischemia time of 19 minutes in the RAPN group versus 25 minutes in the LPN group (P = .03). Kural and colleagues[76] reported a mean warm ischemia time of 27.3 minutes in 11 patients who underwent RAPN, compared with 35.8 minutes in 20 LPN patients (P = .02). Williams and colleagues[79] evaluated 59 LPNs and 27 RAPNs and also reported a lower warm ischemia time for RAPN (18.5 vs 28.0 minutes, P ≤.001), although the authors acknowledge using an early unclamping technique in most of their RAPN cases. Warm ischemia time in multiple RAPN series are presented in **Table 1**.[11,55,57,58,61–72] Studies comparing warm ischemia time of RAPN versus LPN are outlined in **Table 2**.[59,73–79]

Perioperative Outcomes

Initial series by Caruso and colleagues[73] and Deane and colleagues[75] found no differences in operating time or EBL between RAPN and LPN. Similarly, in their matched-pair comparison of 24 patients who underwent either RAPN or LPN, Aron and colleagues[74] reported no differences between the groups in those same operative parameters. Haber and colleagues[78] also found no difference in operating time and LOS in their matched cohort study of 150 patients undergoing RAPN or LPN.

To the contrary, Benway and colleagues[59] reported that RAPN was associated with a significantly decreased EBL (155 vs 196 mL, P = .03) and LOS (2.4 vs 2.7 days, P<.001) compared with LPN. Wang and Bhayani[77] also reported shorter operating time (140 vs 156 minutes, P = .04) and LOS (2.5 vs 2.9 days, P = .03) for RAPN in their series of 40 RAPNs and 62 LPNs. **Table 1** depicts perioperative outcomes of various RAPN series[11,55,57,58,61–72]; studies comparing perioperative outcomes of RAPN versus LPN are outlined in **Table 2**.[59,73–79]

Complications

The overall complication rate can be used to evaluate the safety of new surgical procedures. Nevertheless, as illustrated in a single-surgeon series of LPN by Gill and colleagues,[37] even expert surgeons will continue to refine their surgical techniques, resulting in demonstrable improvements in complication rates despite increasing tumor complexity. Similar improvements are anticipated for RAPN as surgeons progress along the learning curve.

Initial series of RAPN reported complication rates ranging from 0 to 20%.[56] A more recently published multicenter study of 450 consecutive cases of RAPN reported an overall complication rate of 15.8%, including intraoperative and postoperative complications of 1.8% and 14.4%, respectively. Postoperative complications were classified as Clavien grade I–II in 76.1% of cases and grade III–IV in 23.9% of cases. RAPN was converted to OPN or LPN in 0.7% of patients (including a single conversion attributable to robotic malfunction and 2 conversions attributable to persistently positive surgical margins) and to radical nephrectomy in 1.6% of patients. There were no deaths.[83] **Table 1** summarizes complication rates of various RAPN series.[11,55,57,58,61–72]

The postoperative complication rate of 14.4% reported in the multicenter study of 450 RAPN cases by Spana and colleagues[83] compares favorably with the 18.6% postoperative complication rate reported in the 3-institution study of 771 LPN cases by Gill and colleagues.[12] Nevertheless, in the largest comparative study of RAPN to date, Benway and colleagues[59] compared 129 patients and 118 patients who underwent RAPN and LPN, respectively, and reported no significant differences in complication rates between the 2 groups. Series comparing complication rates of RAPN and LPN are presented in **Table 2**.[59,73–79]

Assessing specific complications of RAPN, Spana's multi-institutional analysis found an intraoperative hemorrhage rate of 0.2%. A postoperative hemorrhage rate of 4.9% was reported in the same study.[83] The published postoperative transfusion rates of RAPN range from 3% to 10%, which are comparable with the 5.8% and 3.4% for LPN and OPN, respectively.[56] Although initial urinary leak rates reported for RAPN ranged from 2% to 12.5%,[56] Spana's more contemporary multicenter study of RAPN complications reported a urine leakage rate of 1.6%[83]; these rates are comparable with the 3.1% and 2.3% rates for LPN and OPN, respectively, reported in the multicenter study of 1800 patients by Gill and colleagues.[12]

Taken together, single series[11,55,57,58,61–72] and comparative studies[59,73–79] have found that RAPN can be performed safely and that it is probably not inferior to LPN for the treatment of renal masses in terms of oncologic, functional, and perioperative outcomes. Carefully matched (ideally, randomized) comparisons of OPN, LPN, and RAPN with long-term follow-up are still needed. Recently developed metrics for comparing renal mass complexity (eg, R.E.N.A.L. nephrometry score[84] and PADUA score[85]) may facilitate such comparisons.

SUMMARY

Despite urologists' increasing acceptance of elective partial nephrectomy as a feasible, oncologically sound, and less morbid treatment option for small renal masses, partial nephrectomy remains grossly underutilized, particularly in the community setting. A recent National Cancer database analysis shows that despite increased use of partial nephrectomy, only 47.8% of tumors less than 3 cm diagnosed between 2004 and 2007 were treated with nephron-sparing surgery in the community setting.[2] Factors that may impede the dissemination of partial nephrectomy into general practices include unfounded fears regarding the oncologic efficacy of partial nephrectomy and an underappreciation of the impact of radical nephrectomy on kidney function and overall morbidity and mortality. In the absence of adequate ancillary health services, the greater technical complexity and greater potential for vascular and urinary complications associated with partial nephrectomy, as corroborated in the American Urological Association guidelines,[7] may also deter general urologists from performing this procedure electively. Furthermore, in view of the potential advantages of minimally invasive surgery over open surgery, the high level of expertise required to perform LPN may dissuade some surgeons from performing minimally invasive nephron-sparing surgery in favor of the less technically demanding LRN.

Offering the advantages of LPN in terms of decreased EBL, shorter LOS, improved cosmesis, and more rapid convalescence, while simultaneously helping to surmount some of the technical challenges associated with LPN,[55,75] the emergence of RAPN as a minimally invasive nephron-sparing alternative to LPN may prove crucial in facilitating the wider dissemination of nephron-sparing surgery into general practices. As expertise in robotic surgery has increased, RAPN has been offered to more patients, including those with larger, endophytic, and central masses,[56] and studies have found that RAPN can be performed safely and with acceptable outcomes for increasingly more complex renal tumors.[58,64,69] As a nascent procedure, however, RAPN's ultimate place in general US practices is still being defined. Although comparisons of RAPN and LPN have shown favorable outcomes for RAPN, long-term data on RAPN are still lacking.

The surgical technique for minimally invasive partial nephrectomy continues to evolve. In the next few years, we can expect to see further advances designed to minimize or even eliminate warm ischemia time and facilitate use of cold ischemia during RAPN and LPN. Indeed, some have reported achieving cold ischemia by continuous perfusion of cold isotonic solution through an angiocatheter passed into the main renal artery via a percutaneous femoral puncture.[86] Others have described renal parenchymal hypothermia using retrograde perfusion of the calyceal system with ice-cold saline through a ureteral access sheath.[87] Approaches for implementing cold ischemia in RAPN and LPN via surface irrigation of the kidney with ice-slush, cold saline, and novel cooling substances are also being explored.[88,89]

Technical innovation in robotic instrumentation may enhance the technique of RAPN. For example, precise tumor localization and dissection may be facilitated by the application of systems such as TilePro, which enable picture-on-picture display of radiographic images on the console screen. Use of the fourth robotic arm in the da Vinci S and Si systems decreases the reliance of the surgeon on the bedside assistant during retraction, dissection, and reconstruction. Furthermore, with the advent of robotic bulldog clamps, barbed suture, and the robotic ultrasound probe, the trend for maximizing the autonomy of the console surgeon—particularly during the critical steps of tumor identification, hilar clamping, and renorrhaphy—is becoming increasingly apparent. The future development of robotic systems that can provide tactile feedback to the surgeon may also contribute to the safety and efficacy of RAPN, particularly for complex renal masses.

REFERENCES

1. Kane CJ, Mallin K, Ritchey J, et al. Renal cell cancer stage migration: analysis of the National Cancer Data Base. Cancer 2008;113:78.
2. Cooperberg MR, Mallin K, Kane CJ, et al. Treatment trends for stage I renal cell carcinoma. J Urol 2011;186(2):394.
3. Fergany AF, Hafez KS, Novick AC. Long-term results of nephron sparing surgery for localized renal cell carcinoma: 10-year followup. J Urol 2000;163: 442.
4. Go AS, Chertow GM, Fan D, et al. Chronic kidney disease and the risks of death, cardiovascular events, and hospitalization. N Engl J Med 2004;351:1296.
5. Thompson RH, Boorjian SA, Lohse CM, et al. Radical nephrectomy for pT1a renal masses may be associated with decreased overall survival compared with partial nephrectomy. Cancer 2008;112:511.
6. Weight CJ, Lieser G, Larson BT, et al. Partial nephrectomy is associated with improved overall survival compared to radical nephrectomy in patients with unanticipated benign renal tumors. Eur Urol 2010;58(2):293.
7. Novick AC (Chair), Campbell SC (Co-Chair). American Urological Association Education and Research (AUA) guidelines: Guidelines for management of the clinical stage I renal mass. Renal mass clinical panel chairs. Available at: www.auanet.org/content/media/renalmass09.pdf. Accessed February 23, 2012.
8. Thompson RH, Kaag M, Vickers A, et al. Contemporary use of partial nephrectomy at a tertiary care center in the United States. J Urol 2009;181:993.
9. Clayman RV, Kavoussi LR, Soper NJ, et al. Laparoscopic nephrectomy: initial case report. J Urol 1991;146:278–82.
10. Winfield HN, Donovan JF, Godet AS, et al. Laparoscopic partial nephrectomy: initial case report for benign disease. J Endourol 1993;7:521.
11. Gettman MT, Blute ML, Chow GK, et al. Robot-assisted laparoscopic partial nephrectomy: technique and initial clinical experience with DaVinci robotic system. Urology 2004;64:914.

12. Gill IS, Kavoussi LR, Lane BR, et al. Comparison of 1,800 laparoscopic and open partial nephrectomies for single renal tumors. J Urol 2007;178:41.
13. Lane BR, Gill IS. 7-year oncological outcomes after laparoscopic and open partial nephrectomy. J Urol 2010;183:473.
14. Gill IS, Meraney AM, Schwetzer D. Laparoscopic radical nephrectomy in 100 patients: a single-center experience from the U.S. Cancer 2001;92:1843–55.
15. Hasan WA, Abreu SC, Gill IS. Laparoscopic surgery for renal cell carcinoma. Expert Rev Anticancer Ther 2003;3(6):830–6.
16. Monk TG, Weldon BC. Anesthetic considerations for laparoscopic surgery. J Endurol 1992;6:89.
17. Wolf JS Jr, Clayman RV, McDougall EM, et al. Carbon dioxide and helium insufflation during laparoscopic radical nephrectomy in a patient with severe pulmonary disease. J Urol 1996;155:2021.
18. Weizer AZ, Palella GV, Montgomery JS, et al. Robot-assisted retroperitoneal partial nephrectomy: technique and perioperative results. J Endourol 2011;25:553.
19. Kavoussi LR, Schwartz MJ, Gill IS. Laparoscopic surgery of the kidney. In: Wein AJ, Kavoussi LR, Partin AW, et al, editors. Campbell-Walsh urology. 10th edition. Philadelphia: Saunders, Elsevier Inc; 2011. Chapter 55.
20. Dulabon LM, Stifelman MD. Laparoscopic and robotic partial nephrectomy. Chapter 6. In: Joseph JV, Patel HR, editors. Retroperitoneal robotic and laparoscopic surgery. London: Springer-Verlag; 2011. p. 61.
21. Rogers CG. Retroperitoneal robotic kidney surgery: technique and early results. Available at: http://www.vidoevo.com/yvideo.php?i=alhMUzZCcWuRpZkI4TTQ& retroperitoneal-robotic-kidney-surgery-technique-and-early-results. Accessed February 23, 2012.
22. Tsivian A, Sidi AA. Port site metastases in urological laparoscopic surgery. J Urol 2003;169:1213–8.
23. Cicco A, Salomon L, Hoznek H. Carcinological risks and retroperitoneal laparoscopy. Eur Urol 2000;38:606–12.
24. Kaouk JH, Gill IS. Laparoscopic radical nephrectomy: morcellate or leave intact? Rev Urol 2002;4:38–44.
25. Portis AJ, Yan Y, Landman J. Long-term follow-up after laparoscopic radical nephrectomy. J Urol 2002;167:1257–62.
26. Fentie DD, Barrett PH, Taranger LA. Metastatic renal cell cancer after laparoscopic radical nephrectomy: long-term follow-up. J Endourol 2000;14:407–11.
27. Castillho LN, Fugita OE, Mitre AI. Port site recurrences of renal cell carcinoma after videolaparoscopic radical nephrectomy. J Urol 2001;165:519.
28. Matin FS, Gill IS, Worley S. Outcome of laparoscopic radical and open partial nephrectomy for the sporadic 4 cm or less renal tumor with a normal contralateral kidney. J Urol 2001;168:1356–60.
29. KDOQI clinical practice guidelines for chronic kidney disease: evaluation, classification, and stratification. Available at: http://www.kidney.org/professionals/ KDOQI/guidelines_ckd/toc.htm. Accessed February 22, 2012.
30. Huang WC, Levey AS, Serio AM, et al. Chronic kidney disease after nephrectomy in patients with renal cortical tumors: a retrospective cohort study. Lancet Oncol 2006;7:735–40.
31. Steinberg AP, Desai MM, Kaouk JH. The large (>7 cm; pT2) renal tumor: laparoscopic versus open radical nephrectomy. J Endourol 2002;16:A160.
32. Steinberg AP, Finelli A, Desai MM, et al. Laparoscopic radical nephrectomy for large (greater than 7 cm, T2) renal tumors. J Urol 2004;172(6):2172–6.

33. Cha EK, Wiklund NP, Scherr DS, et al. Recent advances in robot-assisted radical cystectomy. Curr Opin Urol 2011;21:65.
34. Siqueira TM, Kuo RL, Gardner TA. Major complications in 213 laparoscopic nephrectomy cases: the Indianapolis experience. J Urol 2002;168:1361-5.
35. Becker F, Van Poppel H, Hakenberg OW, et al. Assessing the impact of ischemia time during partial nephrectomy. Eur Urol 2009;56:625.
36. Thompson RH, Lane BR, Lohse CM, et al. Every minute counts when the renal hilum is clamped during partial nephrectomy. Eur Urol 2010;58:340.
37. Gill IS, Kamoi K, Aron M, et al. 800 laparoscopic partial nephrectomies: a single surgeon series. J Urol 2010;183:34.
38. Benway BM, Baca G, Bhayani SB, et al. Selective versus nonselective arterial clamping during laparoscopic partial nephrectomy: impact upon renal function in the setting of a solitary kidney in a porcine model. J Endourol 2009;23: 1127-33.
39. Figenshau RS. Laparoscopic partial nephrectomy with segmental renal vascular control. J Endourol 2005;19(Suppl 1):A257.
40. Gill IS, Eisenberg MS, Aron M, et al. 'Zero ischemia' partial nephrectomy: novel laparoscopic and robotic technique. Eur Urol 2011;59:128.
41. Bhayani SB, Rha KH, Pinto PA, et al. Laparoscopic partial nephrectomy: effect of warm ischemia time on serum creatinine. J Urol 2004;172:1264.
42. Foyil KV, Ames CD, Ferguson GG, et al. Long-term changes in creatinine clearance after laparoscopic renal surgery. J Am Coll Surg 2007;206:511.
43. Canales BK, Lynch AC, Fernandes E, et al. Novel technique of knotless hemostatic renal parenchymal suture repair during laparoscopic partial nephrectomy. Urology 2007;70(2):358-9.
44. Hollenback BK, Taub DA, Miller DC, et al. National utilization trends of partial nephrectomy for renal cell carcinoma: a case of underutilization? Urology 2006; 67:254.
45. Kaouk JH, Gill IS. Laparoscopic partial nephrectomy: a new horizon. Curr Opin Urol 2003;13(3):215-9.
46. Desai MM, Gill IS, Kaouk JH. Laparoscopic partial nephrectomy with suture-repair of the collecting system. Urology 2003;61:99-104.
47. Gill IS, Matin SF, Desai MM, et al. Comparative analysis of laparoscopic versus open partial nephrectomy for renal tumors in 200 patients. J Urol 2003;170(1): 64-8.
48. Gill IS, Desai MM, Kaouk JH. Laparoscopic partial nephrectomy for renal tumor: duplicating open surgical techniques. J Urol 2002;167:469-76.
49. Rassweiler JJ, Abbou C, Janetschek G, et al. Laparoscopic partial nephrectomy. The European experience. Urol Clin North Am 2000;27:721-36.
50. Cabello JM, Bhayani SB, Figenshau RS, et al. Camera and trocar placement for robot-assisted radical and partial nephrectomy: which configuration provides optimal visualization and instrument mobility? J Robotic Surg 2009;3:155.
51. Bhayani SB, Figensha RS. The Washington University renorrhaphy for robotic partial nephrectomy: a detailed description of the technique displayed at the 2008 World Robotic Urologic Symposium. J Robotic Surg 2008;2:139-40.
52. Benway BM, Wang AJ, Cabello JM, et al. Robotic partial nephrectomy with sliding-clip renorrhaphy: technique and outcomes. Eur Urol 2009;55:592.
53. Sukumar S, Rogers CG. Robotic partial nephrectomy: surgical technique. BJU Int 2011;108:942.
54. Sammon J, Petros F, Sukumar, et al. Barbed suture for renorrhaphy during robot-assisted partial nephrectomy. J Endourol 2011;25:529.

55. Mottrie A, De Naeyer G, Schatteman P, et al. Impact of the learning curve on peri-operative outcomes in patients who underwent robotic partial nephrectomy for parenchymal renal tumors. Eur Urol 2010;58:127.
56. Cha EK, Lee DJ, Del Pizzo JJ. Current status of robotic partial nephrectomy (RPN). BJU Int 2011;108:935.
57. Scoll BJ, Uzzo RG, Chen DY, et al. Robot-assisted partial nephrectomy: a large single-institutional experience. Urology 2010;75:1328.
58. Dulabon LM, Kaouk JH, Haber GP, et al. Multi-institutional analysis of robotic partial nephrectomy for hilar versus nonhilar lesions in 446 consecutive cases. Eur Urol 2011;59:325.
59. Benway BM, Bhayni SB, Rogers CG, et al. Robot-assisted partial nephrectomy versus laparoscopic partial nephrectomy for renal tumors: a multi-institutional analysis of peri-operative outcomes. J Urol 2009;182:866.
60. Benway BM, Bhayani SB. Surgical outcomes of robot-assisted partial nephrectomy. BJU Int 2011;108:955.
61. Phillips CK, Taneja SS, Stifelman M. Robot-assisted laparoscopic partial nephrectomy: the NYU technique. J Endourol 2005;19:441.
62. Kaul S, Laungani R, Sarle R. da Vinci-assisted robotic partial nephrectomy: technique and results at a mean of 15 months of follow-up. Eur Urol 2007;51:186.
63. Bhayani SB, Das N. Robotic assisted laparoscopic partial nephrectomy for suspected renal cell carcinoma: retrospective review of surgical outcomes of 35 cases. BMC Surg 2008;8:16.
64. Rogers CG, Metwalli A, Blatt AM, et al. Robotic partial nephrectomy for renal hilar tumors: a multi-institutional analysis. J Urol 2008;180:2353.
65. Ho H, Schwentner C, Neururer R, et al. Robot-assisted laparoscopic partial nephrectomy: surgical technique and clinical outcomes at 1 year. BJU Int 2009;103:663–8.
66. Michli EE, Parra RO. Robot-assisted laparoscopic partial nephrectomy: initial clinical experience. Urology 2009;73:302–5.
67. Gong Y, Du C, Josephson DY, et al. Four-arm robotic partial nephrectomy for complex renal cell carcinoma. World J Urol 2010;28:111–5.
68. Benway BM, Bhayani SB, Rogers CG, et al. Robot-assisted partial nephrectomy: an international experience. Eur Urol 2010;57:815.
69. Patel MN, Krane LS, Bhandari, et al. Robotic partial nephrectomy for renal tumors larger than 4 cm. Eur Urol 2010;57:310.
70. Petros FG, Patel MN, Kheterpal E, et al. Robotic partial nephrectomy in the setting of prior abdominal surgery. BJU Int 2011;108:413.
71. Lorenzo EI, Jeong W, Oh CK, et al. Robotics applied in laparoscopic kidney surgery. The Yonsei University experience of 127 cases. Urology 2011;77:114.
72. Naeem N, Petros F, Sukumar S, et al. Robot-assisted partial nephrectomy in obese patients. J Endourol 2011;25:101.
73. Caruso RP, Phillips CK, Kau E, et al. Robot-assisted laparoscopic partial nephrectomy: initial experience. J Urol 2006;176:36.
74. Aron M, Koenig P, Kaouk JH, et al. Robotic and laparoscopic partial nephrectomy: a matched-pair comparison from a high-volume center. BJU Int 2008; 102:86.
75. Deane LA, Lee HJ, Box GN, et al. Robotic versus standard laparoscopic partial/wedge nephrectomy: a comparison of intraoperative and perioperative results from a single institution. J Endourol 2008;22:947.
76. Kural AR, Atug F, Tufek I, et al. Robot-assisted partial nephrectomy versus laparoscopic partial nephrectomy: comparison of outcomes. J Endourol 2009;23:1491.

77. Wang AJ, Bhayani SB. Robotic partial nephrectomy versus laparoscopic partial nephrectomy for renal cell carcinoma: single-surgeon analysis of >100 consecutive procedures. Urology 2009;73:306.
78. Haber GP, White WM, Crouzet S, et al. Robotic versus laparoscopic partial nephrectomy: single-surgeon matched cohort study of 150 patients. Urology 2010;76:754.
79. Williams SB, Kacker R, Alemozaffar M, et al. Robotic partial nephrectomy versus laparoscopic partial nephrectomy: a single laparoscopic trained surgeon's experience in the development of a robotic partial nephrectomy program. World J Urol 2011. [Epub ahead of print]. http://dx.doi.org/10.1007/s00345-011-0648-5.
80. Kwon EO, Carver BS, Snyder ME, et al. Impact of positive surgical margins in patients undergoing partial nephrectomy for renal cortical tumors. BJU Int 2007;99:286.
81. Sundaram V, Figenshau RS, Roytman TM, et al. Positive margin during partial nephrectomy: does cancer remain in the renal remnant? Urology 2011;77:1400.
82. Porpiglia F, Volpe A, Billia M, et al. Laparoscopic versus open partial nephrectomy: analysis of the current literature. Eur Urol 2008;53:732.
83. Spana G, Haber GP, Dulabon LM, et al. Complications after robotic partial nephrectomy at centers of excellence: multi-institutional analysis of 450 cases. J Urol 2011;186:417.
84. Kutikov A, Uzzo RG. The R.E.N.A.L. nephrometry score: a comprehensive standardized system for quantitating renal tumor size, location, and depth. J Urol 2009;182:844.
85. Ficarra V, Novara G, Secco S, et al. Preoperative aspects and dimensions used for anatomical (PADU) classification of renal tumors in patients who are candidates for nephron-sparing surgery. Eur Urol 2009;56:786.
86. Hermann TR, Kruck S, Nagele U. Transperitoneal in situ intraarterial cooling in laparoscopic partial nephrectomy. World J Urol 2011;29:337.
87. Landman J, Rehman J, Sundaram CP, et al. Renal hypothermia achieved by retrograde intra-cavitary saline perfusion. J Enourol 2002;16(7):445.
88. Kijvikai K, Viprakasit DP, Milhoua P, et al. A simple, effective method to create laparoscopic renal protective hypothermia with cold saline surface irrigation: clinical application and assessment. J Urol 2010;184:1861.
89. Schoeppler G, Klippstein E, Hell J, et al. Prolonged cold ischemia for laparoscopic partial nephrectomy with a new cooling material: freka-Gelice- a comparison of four cooling methods. J Endourol 2010;24:1151.

Laparoscopic Adrenalectomy for Cancer

Jennifer Creamer, MD[a], Brent D. Matthews, MD[b],*

KEYWORDS

- Laparoscopy • Minimally invasive surgery • Adrenal metastases • Incidentaloma
- Adrenal malignancy

KEY POINTS

- Although an incidental adrenal mass is likely to be benign, a surgeon should be capable of coordinating the diagnostic evaluation.
- Adrenalectomy is warranted for all lesions suspected to be adrenal cortical carcinoma and for nonmalignant masses that are metabolically active.
- There is no consensus on the use of laparoscopy in adrenal malignancy. Studies have shown that a laparoscopic approach can be an acceptable option for primary neoplasms and adrenal metastases with no evidence of local invasion.

INTRODUCTION

Laparoscopy has become a widely accepted technical platform in nearly all areas of surgery since its introduction with laparoscopic cholecystectomy in the late 1980s. First introduced by Gagner and colleagues in 1992 for patients with Cushing syndrome and pheochromocytoma, laparoscopic adrenalectomy has gained acceptance for management of most benign tumors including aldosteronomas and adrenal incidentalomas. Laparoscopic adrenalectomy results in fewer perioperative complications, decreased postoperative pain and hospital stay, and more effective use of health care expenditures.[1,2] It has been reported to be less morbid, more cost-effective, and to allow patients to recover faster compared with an open approach.[3,4] Controversy remains regarding laparoscopic adrenalectomy for large tumors and malignant

Disclosure: The material contained herein has not been previously published or submitted elsewhere for publication and will not be sent to another journal until a decision is made concerning publication by the *Surgical Oncology Clinics of North America*. In addition, the authors cite no personal conflicts of interest or financial arrangements with the organizations, corporations, and/or devices detailed in this article. No sources of external funding were used.

[a] Department of General Surgery, William Beaumont Army Medical Center, 5005 North Piedras, El Paso, TX 79920, USA; [b] Section of Minimally Invasive Surgery, Department of Surgery, Washington University School of Medicine, 660 South Euclid Avenue, Box 8109, St Louis, MO 63110, USA
* Corresponding author.
E-mail address: matthewsbr@wustl.edu

or potentially malignant adrenal lesions. This article reviews the latest trends in laparoscopic surgery for adrenalectomy in malignant adrenal tumors.

INCIDENTAL ADRENAL MASS

The discovery of an incidental adrenal mass has become increasingly common with the routine use of computed tomography (CT) scans for diagnostic evaluations of abdominal pain, cancer screening, and other unrelated complaints. Adrenal incidentalomas, defined as any adrenal mass 1 cm or more in diameter discovered on a radiologic examination performed for indications other than adrenal disease, have become a common finding on CT scans, with reported rates from 0.8% to 5% (**Fig. 1**).[5] This rate is consistent with autopsy reports showing a mean prevalence of 2.3%.[6] The prevalence of adrenal incidentalomas increases with age, being seen in less than 1% of patients younger than 30 years compared with 6.9% in those older than 70 years.[7] The differential diagnosis of an incidentaloma includes benign lesions such as adrenal adenoma, adrenal cyst, pheochromocytoma, myelolipoma, ganglioneuroma, or hematoma, but must also include malignant lesions such as adrenal cortical carcinoma (ACC), malignant pheochromocytoma, or metastatic disease from a nonadrenal primary source. Although likely benign, a surgeon should be capable of coordinating the diagnostic evaluation of an incidental adrenal mass to establish tumor functionality, malignant potential, and indications for resection (hormonal and radiological work-up are discussed later).

Adrenalectomy is warranted for all lesions suspected to be ACCs, and for nonmalignant masses that are metabolically active. If a unilateral incidentaloma is found to be biochemically active, laparoscopic adrenalectomy is the treatment of choice after appropriate preoperative preparation such as α blockade for pheochromocytoma to prevent perioperative hypertensive crisis. Adrenal tumors considered to be an ACC should be resected. The specific surgical approach is discussed later in more detail.

In patients with a nonfunctioning adrenal mass, the size of the incidentaloma is the major determinant of which therapy is indicated. A lesion greater than 6 cm should be resected, because 25% are ACC. In contrast, greater than 98% of incidentalomas less than 4 cm are benign. If an adrenal incidentaloma is less than 4 cm and deemed low risk by imaging criteria, there is no absolute indication for resection.[8] Repeat imaging

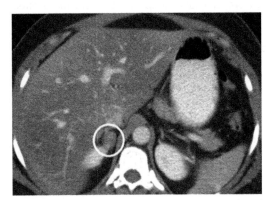

Fig. 1. Contrast-enhanced CT of the abdomen showed a 2.2-cm right adrenal incidentaloma (*circle*; 55–80 Hounsfield units). Biochemical evaluation showed subclinical Cushing syndrome. Laparoscopic resection and pathologic examination confirmed the diagnosis of adrenal cortical adenoma. (*From* Bittner JG 4th, Brunt LM. Evaluation and management of adrenal incidentaloma. J Surg Oncol 2012;106(5):557–64; with permission.)

should be performed in 6 to 12 months. If the size remains unchanged, no further follow-up is indicated. Enlargement of greater than 1 cm in 1 year requires short-interval follow-up or consideration for adrenalectomy.[9] Approximately 6% of adrenal lesions between 4 and 6 cm are malignant. Therefore, laparoscopic adrenalectomy is recommended in appropriate surgical candidates. Nevertheless, repeat CT scan and nonoperative observation is an option in high-risk surgical patients who have comorbidities potentially complicating elective surgery. Imaging characteristics that suggest anything other than a benign adenoma or rapid growth (>1 cm in 1 year) on repeat imaging at intervals of 3 to 6 months should be managed with adrenalectomy.[9] Lesions less than 4 cm can be resected with special consideration to patient age, ability of patient to comply with radiographic follow-up, and surgeon expertise with laparoscopic adrenalectomy.

Evaluation of Hormone Function

The diagnostic evaluation of an adrenal incidentaloma requires a biochemical evaluation for hormonal activity. The most cost-effective evaluation of an adrenal incidentaloma includes a serum potassium, low-dose dexamethasone suppression test, and plasma metanephrines. If a patient is hypokalemic, plasma aldosterone and renin levels should be determined. A plasma aldosterone/renin activity ratio greater than 30 with plasma aldosterone concentration greater than 5 nmol/L (20 ng/dL) suggests autonomous aldosterone activity. An increase in plasma metanephrines has a sensitivity of 99% and specificity of 89% for pheochromocytoma. A low-dose overnight dexamethasone suppression test is used to screen for hypercortisolism. After a patient is given 1 mg of dexamethasone at 11 PM the night before an 8 AM serum cortisol blood sample, normal individuals exhibit a suppressed serum cortisol level to less than 139 nmol/L (5 μg/dL). Should the cortisol level fail to suppress appropriately after low-dose dexamethasone administration, 24-hour urine-free cortisol or salivary cortisol testing should be done to confirm the diagnosis.[8,10] If hypercortisolism is confirmed, an adrenocorticotropic hormone (ACTH) level should be obtained. ACTH levels are suppressed in adrenal Cushing syndrome and normal or increased in ACTH-independent Cushing syndrome.[11]

Radiologic Evaluation

The most common radiologic imaging for adrenal mass is CT scan or magnetic resonance imaging (MRI). Benign adrenal adenomas appear as a homogeneous smooth mass and typically have an attenuation value less than 10 Hounsfield units (HU). Adrenal lesions with an attenuation value of greater than 10 HU in an unenhanced CT scan or enhancement washout of less than 50% and a delayed attenuation of greater than 35 HU (on 10-minute to 15-minute delayed enhanced CT scan) are suspicious for malignancy.[12–17] Adrenocortical carcinomas (ACCs) are frequently large (>6 cm), appear heterogeneous, with irregular borders and focal areas of hemorrhage and necrosis.[18] Local invasion or tumor extension into the inferior vena cava, as well as lymph node or distant metastases (lung and liver), are frequently found in advanced ACC. Adrenal metastases often occur in the setting of other metastatic disease, they are usually higher in attenuation, and may have irregular borders.[11]

Adenomas have an intensity similar to liver on T2-weighted MRI. However, T2-weighted MRI for pheochromocytomas has a characteristic bright appearance caused by an increased uptake of labeled noradrenaline analogues ^{123}I-meta-iodobenzylguanidine and ^{131}I-meta-iodobenzylguanidine.[12] Invasion into adjacent organs and into the inferior vena cava is best determined with MRI.

A small proportion of adrenal incidentalomas remain indeterminate after CT and/or MRI. With a history of malignancy and an isolated adrenal mass, positron emission tomography (PET)/CT may be considered. If PET/CT is performed, most malignant lesions show avidity for ^{18}F-fluorodeoxyglucose and most benign lesions do not.[11]

Needle biopsy has a limited role in the evaluation of adrenal incidentaloma. In general, fine-needle aspiration (FNA) biopsy is not useful in the diagnostic work-up of patients with incidentally discovered adrenal masses and rarely alters management in patients with resectable adrenal metastases and primary adrenal malignancies.[19] The complications of adrenal FNA, such as pneumothorax, bleeding, hypertensive crisis, and needle-track metastasis, need to be considered before performing this procedure.[8,20,21] The indications for FNA biopsy are suspected infection or adrenal metastasis in the setting of other extra-adrenal metastatic disease.[11]

MALIGNANT ADRENAL GLAND TUMORS
Malignant Pheochromocytoma

Pheochromocytomas are rare catecholamine-secreting tumors derived from chromaffin cells, with an incidence of 1 to 2/100,000 adults per year.[22] Between 5% and 26% of pheochromocytomas are malignant and they are more likely to be malignant if there is a family history of malignant pheochromocytoma.[23–27] Despite multiple laparoscopically resected pheochromocytomas reported in the current literature, there is a lack of data on the long-term follow-up of patients who have undergone laparoscopic adrenalectomy for malignant pheochromocytoma. Following open resection, patients have a variable disease-free survival because malignant pheochromocytoma may recur early or even more than 20 years after the initial resection.[24–34] For this reason, it may be impossible to detect a difference in recurrence compared with a laparoscopic adrenalectomy. A randomized prospective trial comparing the 2 methods is unlikely considering the rarity of malignant pheochromocytoma and the difficulty in accurately diagnosing malignancy before surgery.

ACC

ACCs are rare, with an incidence of 1 to 2 per million.[22,35,36] ACCs make up about 5% of all adrenal incidentilomas.[6] They have a bimodal age distribution with peak incidences in early childhood and the fourth to fifth decades of life, with a female/male prevalence ratio of 1.5:1.[37,38] Most cases are sporadic, but ACCs can be associated with several hereditary syndromes including Li-Fraumeni syndrome, Beckwith-Wiedemann syndrome, and multiple endocrine neoplasia type 1 (MEN 1).[39–43] Although the underlying mechanism of carcinogenesis in sporadic ACCs has yet to be fully determined, inactivating somatic mutations of the p53 tumor suppressor gene (chromosome 17p13) and alterations at the 11p15 locus (site of the IGF-2 gene) seem to frequently occur.[44–47]

At presentation, about 60% of patients have evidence of adrenal steroid hormone excess, with or without virilization.[22,48–50] In addition to the standard work-up for an incidentaloma, tumors determined to be biochemically active may require further testing; 24-hour fractionate catecholamines and urine total metanephrine levels should be performed in patients with signs of a pheochromocytoma such as tachycardia, severe hypertension, cardiac palpitations or arrhythmias, anxiety, and sweating. Those exhibiting signs and symptoms associated with hypersecretion of cortisol (Cushing syndrome), including weight gain, weakness, hypertension, psychiatric disturbances, hirsutism, centripetal obesity, purple striae, buffalo hump, supraclavicular fat pad enlargement, hyperglycemia, and hypokalemia, should be evaluated with 24-hour urinary excretion of cortisol and ACTH levels.[48] Androgen-secreting tumors in women may induce hirsutism, deepening of the voice, and oligomenorrhea/amenorrhea. In men, estrogen-secreting tumors may induce gyneco-mastia and testicular atrophy. The clinical diagnosis of adrenal-induced virilization can be confirmed by measuring serum testosterone, serum adrenal androgens (dehydroe-piandrosterone [DHEA] and DHEA-sulfate) and 24-hour 17-ketosteroid.[51] Aldoste-rone-secreting tumors can be evaluated by measuring serum potassium, plasma aldosterone concentration, and plasma renin activity; they may present with hyperten-sion, weakness, and hypokalemia. ACCs that are hormonally inactive typically present with symptoms related to tumor burden, including abdominal pain, back pain, early satiety, and weight loss.[48,52] ACCs are typically large with irregular borders on CT **(Fig. 2)**.[53] Most ACCs are greater than 6 cm at presentation; however, ACCs smaller than 6 cm have been increasingly reported.[35] Distant metastasis is present in 20% to 50% of cases on diagnosis.[54–57]

The overall prognosis for ACC is poor, with 5-year survival rates less than 40%.[22,35,58] Even in patients who undergo complete operative resection, recurrence is common. Around two-thirds of patients develop recurrence within 2 years of treat-ment and 85% of patients develop local recurrence or distant metastases.[57,59]

Treatment of nonmetastatic adrenal carcinoma

Long-term survival in ACCs is determined by tumor stage at presentation and curative resection by an experienced surgeon.[22] In patients with localized ACCs, surgical resection of the tumor with removal of adjacent lymph nodes is recommended, which may require removal of adjacent structures such as the liver, kidney, pancreas, spleen, and/or diaphragm for complete resections. Performing an aggressive oncologic resection has limited the application of laparoscopy for these locally invasive tumors. Therefore, at this time the decision between open and laparoscopic resection for ACCs or tumors with a high risk of being malignant remains controversial. Neverthe-less, the indications for open adrenalectomy have recently been challenged given the increased experience with laparoscopic adrenalectomy. Recent reports have shown acceptable oncologic outcomes following laparoscopic adrenalectomy for

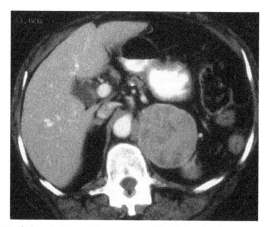

Fig. 2. Enhanced CT of the abdomen for nonspecific abdominal pain revealed an irregular-shaped, heterogeneous, and calcified left adrenal mass. On pathologic examination, the mass turned out to be an adrenocortical carcinoma. (*From* Bittner JG 4th, Brunt LM. Evalu-ation and management of adrenal incidentaloma. J Surg Oncol 2012;106(5):557–64; with permission.)

early-stage adrenocortical carcinoma but the overall oncologic effectiveness of laparoscopic adrenalectomy for the resection of ACCs remains unclear.

Open versus laparoscopic adrenalectomy for ACCs

Because of the rarity of ACC, studies comparing the efficacy of laparoscopic adrenalectomy versus open adrenalectomy are limited. Reported data are limited by several factors, including small patient populations, being retrospective in nature, and having limited or no follow-up. Advocates for open adrenalectomy contend that laparoscopic adrenalectomy limits the ability to adhere to oncologic principles of resection. Examples include insufficient tactile sensation, limited tumor retraction, and difficult retroperitoneal fat resection. These limitations can lead to rupture of the capsule and spread of tumor cells from unrecognized microscopic extensions of the tumor in the operative field.[60]

Early use of laparoscopic adrenalectomy for ACC

Early case reports showed poor outcomes with the use of laparoscopic adrenalectomy. Between 1997 and 1999, case reports describe 5 patients who developed disease recurrence within 4 to 14 months. Recurrences were manifested locally, at port-sites, or as diffuse carcinomatosis.[61–65] Outcomes have since improved and a review of 11 case series including 48 cases of primary ACC from 2002 to 2007 showed comparable rates of recurrence in laparoscopic adrenalectomy compared with open adrenalectomy performed for primary adrenal malignancy.[66] Only 1 series reported peritoneal carcinomatosis in 5 patients undergoing laparoscopic adrenalectomy (all referred patients) and there was 1 report of port-site recurrence.[67,68] Although outcomes were similar to those of open adrenalectomy, the series were lacking in case volume, with only 2 to 13 patients with ACC per series, and long-term follow-up was not reported.

Recent use of laparoscopic adrenalectomy for ACC

In 2010, 4 retrospective studies were published comparing laparoscopic adrenalectomy with open adrenalectomy for ACC; 2 showed equivalent oncologic results, whereas the other 2 showed worse outcomes in patients who underwent laparoscopic adrenalectomy (**Table 1**).[69–72] Porpilgia and colleagues[69] showed no significant difference in recurrence-free survival between patients with stage 1 and 2 ACC in 18 patients who underwent laparoscopic adrenalectomy compared with 25 who underwent open adrenalectomy. This study was limited by its short follow-up and exclusion

Table 1
Summary of retrospective 2010 studies

Author (Reference)	Number of Patients	Mean/Median Follow-up (mo)	Recurrence (%)	Mean/Median Time to Recurrence (mo)	Peritoneal Carcinomatosis
Brix et al,[70] 2010	117 OA 35 LA	32 OA 64 LA	81 (69) OA 27 (77) LA	NR	—
Miller et al,[72] 2010	71 OA 17 LA	36.5	(65) OA (63) LA	19.2 OA 9.6 LA	—
Leboulleux et al,[71] 2010	58 OA 6 LA	35	NR	NR	4-y rate 27% OA 67% LA
Porpiglia et al,[69] 2010	25 OA 18 LA	38 OA 30 LA	16 (64) OA 9 (50) LA	18 OA 23 LA	—

Abbreviations: LA, laparoscopic adrenalectomy; OA, open adrenalectomy.

of patients who did not have radical resections or who had macroscopically incomplete resection, tumor capsule violation, conversion from laparoscopic to open surgery, and those found to have microscopic periadrenal fat invasion on final pathology. Brix and colleagues[70] reached a similar conclusion and suggested that laparoscopic adrenalectomy performed by an experienced surgeon is justified for potentially malignant adrenal incidentalomas and for selected cases of stage I and II ACC. They reported no difference in survival, disease-free recurrence, tumor capsule violation, or peritoneal carcinomatosis between 117 patients undergoing open adrenalectomy and 35 patients undergoing laparoscopic adrenalectomy for stage 1 to 3 ACCs of less than 10 cm. Again, limitations include small sample sizes and limited follow-up in some patients. In 12/35 patients, laparoscopic adrenalectomy was converted to open adrenalectomy because of bleeding (n = 4), adhesions (n = 4), bowel perforation (n = 1), or other technical problems (n = 2).[70]

Leboulleux and colleagues[71] and Miller and colleagues[72] described dissimilar results for laparoscopic adrenalectomy for ACC. Leboulleux and colleagues[71] sought to identify whether the surgical approach in ACC was a risk factor of peritoneal carcinomatosis. They reviewed 64 patients with stages 1 to 4 disease; 58 who underwent open adrenalectomy and 6 who underwent laparoscopic adrenalectomy. Peritoneal carcinomatosis occurred in 18 patients, with a 4-year rate of peritoneal carcinomatosis of 67% for laparoscopic adrenalectomy and 27% for open adrenalectomy. The only risk factor identified was the surgical approach. Miller and colleagues[72] performed a retrospective review comparing 17 patients undergoing laparoscopic adrenalectomy and 71 undergoing open adrenalectomy for ACC. None of the patients in their series underwent laparoscopic adrenalectomy at their institution. Patients who had laparoscopic adrenalectomy had significantly faster local recurrence in the tumor bed, a significantly higher incidence of violation of the tumor capsule, positive margins at resection, and great rates of peritoneal recurrence. Overall recurrence was similar in both groups: 63% in the laparoscopic group and 65% in the open group. Based on their results, Miller and colleagues[72] stated that laparoscopic resection in ACC is inappropriate and should not be attempted.

There is currently no consensus opinion on the role of laparoscopic adrenalectomy in ACC. The 2012 National Comprehensive Cancer Network (NCCN) guidelines advocate the use of open adrenalectomy for ACC because of the potential increased risk for local recurrence and peritoneal spread that has been reported with laparoscopic adrenalectomy. [9,73,74] At a debate on laparoscopic versus open adrenalectomy, advocates for laparoscopic adrenalectomy at the third International Adrenal Cancer Symposium suggested that laparoscopic adrenalectomy can be considered if it can be performed at a referral center and be extracted without fragmentation.[60] If these 2 criteria can be fulfilled, the laparoscopy can be performed on small incidentalomas, indeterminate large incidentalomas without necrosis or evidence of invasion, and small ACCs.[60] Because of the rarity of ACC, a randomized prospective study comparing open with laparoscopic adrenalectomy is unlikely.

Debate will continue to ensue until a consensus opinion is made. If laparoscopic adrenalectomy is performed for ACC, strict oncologic principles must be applied with early consideration for conversion to open adrenalectomy. The use of flexible laparoscopic ultrasound probes has proved to be helpful in cases of laparoscopic adrenalectomy. It can serve as a way to restore the haptic sense that is inherently reduced in laparoscopic surgery. Several investigators have endorsed their use during surgery to identify the adrenal gland and adrenal vein, determine laparoscopic respectability of large adrenal tumors, and to define the line of transection in cases in which only a partial adrenalectomy is performed.[75,76] In addition, techniques like wound protectors, evacuation of the pneumoperitoneum through the port, and perito-neal wound closure have been proposed and applied successfully, but without validation.[77–80]

Metastasis to the Adrenal Gland

Solitary adrenal metastases are common and normally do not cause symptoms. The primary location of a metastatic tumor is most commonly the lung. Additional tumor primaries include breast, kidney, colon, stomach, lymphoma, and melanoma. In patients with known malignancy there is a 45% to 73% chance that their adrenal inci-dentaloma is a metastasis.[81–83] With the increased use of imaging technologies (CT, MRI, PET) the detection of metastases is becoming increasingly common and makes up around 2.1% of adrenal incidentalomas (**Fig. 3**).[6,84]

Treatment of metastasis to the adrenal gland

Resection of isolated metachronous adrenal metastases from various primary cancers may improve survival. Studies have shown a median survival between 20 and 30 months after adrenal metastasectomy, compared with 6 to 8 months in cases without resection.[85,86] In most cases, adrenal metastases are confined within the capsule, suggesting that laparoscopic adrenalectomy may be adequate to achieve negative margins.[32,87]

Open versus laparoscopic adrenalectomy for solitary adrenal metastases

Similar debates to that concerning ACC can be found regarding the approach for resection of solitary adrenal metastases. Concerns have been raised over port-site recurrence. Although most series have not reported port-site recurrences, there have been isolated case reports documenting port-site recurrence after laparoscopic adrenalectomy.[88–91]

Oncologic results comparing laparoscopic adrenalectomy with open adrenalec-tomy have been promising (**Table 2**). Adler and colleagues[92] performed a retrospective review comparing 9 patients who underwent laparoscopic adrenalectomy for adrenal metastases with 8 patients who underwent open adrenalectomy. With a follow-up of 97 months (mean 19 months laparoscopic and 17 months open), they found no port-site metastases, no tumor recurrences, and no difference in survival between the 2 groups. Strong and colleagues[93] compared the results of 31 laparoscopic and 63 open adrenalectomies performed for adrenal metastases. There were no differences

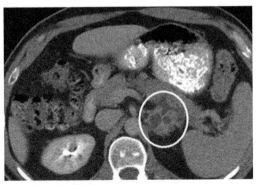

Fig. 3. Enhanced CT of the abdomen for metastatic work-up showed an irregular-shaped, heterogeneous, and high-attenuation left adrenal mass (*circle*) consistent with adrenal metastasis. (*From* Bittner JG 4th, Brunt LM. Evaluation and management of adrenal inciden-taloma. J Surg Oncol 2012;106(5):557–64; with permission.)

Table 2
Series with comparison between open and laparoscopic adrenalectomy for adrenal metastases

Authors	Year	Number of Patients	Mean/Median Follow-up (mo)	Mean/Median Survival (mo)	5-y Survival	Notes on 5-y Survival
Sarela et al[87]	2003	30 OA 11 LA	16	28 OA NR LA	29%[a] LA	—
Adler et al[92]	2007	8 OA 9 LA	12 OA 13 LA	17 OA 19 LA	54% OA 34% LA	No significant difference in 5-y survival
Strong et al[93]	2007	63 OA[b] 31 LA[b]	62 OA 22 LA	30 OA 31 LA	32% OA 29% LA	No significant difference in 5-y survival[c]
Muth et al[95]	2010	20 OA 10 LA	22 OA 18 LA	46 OA 20 LA	22.5%[a]	No significant difference in 5-y survival

[a] Pooled calculation without specific group comparison.
[b] Some patients included in previous series by Sarela and colleagues.[87]
[c] In subset analysis including all tumors less than 4.5 cm (n = 24 LA and n = 25 OA).

in the positive margin rate between a laparoscopic (22%) versus an open (29%) technique, and the median survival for the groups was similar (approximately 30 months). They also showed that the laparoscopic group benefited from a decrease in blood loss, shorter operative time, shorter hospital stay, and decreased complication rates. Other investigators reporting retrospective data on laparoscopic adrenalectomy have shown no differences in the incidence of positive resection margins or survival with similar groups undergoing open resection of adrenal metastases.[87,94,95]

Although the surgical technique to resect adrenal metastases remains controversial, a consensus statement was made at the 2011 Workshop of the European Society of Endocrine Surgeons. It was concluded that a patient with suspected adrenal metastasis should be considered a candidate for adrenalectomy when (1) control of extra-adrenal disease can be accomplished, (2) metastasis is isolated to the adrenal gland(s), (3) adrenal imaging strongly suggests metastasis or the patient has a biopsy-proven adrenal malignancy, (4) metastasis is confined to the adrenal gland as assessed by a recent imaging study, and (5) the patient's performance status warrants an aggressive approach. It was also concluded that, in properly selected patients, laparoscopic (or retroperitoneoscopic) adrenalectomy is a feasible and safe option.[96]

SUMMARY

There is currently no consensus on the use of laparoscopy in adrenal malignancy. Studies have shown that a laparoscopic approach is an acceptable option for primary neoplasms and adrenal metastases with no evidence of local invasion. Nevertheless, in patients who prove to have local invasion during surgery, the laparoscopic approach should be converted to open procedure to allow for a curative wide radical resection.

REFERENCES

1. Brunt LM. The positive impact of laparoscopic adrenalectomy on complications of adrenal surgery. Surg Endosc 2002;16(2):252–7.

2. Brunt LM. Minimal access adrenal surgery. Surg Endosc 2006;20(3):351–61.
3. Kercher KW, Novitsky YW, Park AP, et al. Laparoscopic curative resection of pheochromocytomas. Ann Surg 2005;241(6):919–26.
4. Assalia A, Gagner M. Adrenalectomy. In: Assalia A, Gagner M, Schein M, editors. Controversies in laparoscopic surgery. Berlin, Heidelberg (Germany): Springer; 2006. p. 315–56.
5. Davenport C, Liew A, Doherty B, et al. The prevalence of adrenal incidentaloma in routine clinical practice. Endocrine 2011;40:80–3.
6. Barzon L, Sonino N, Fallo F, et al. Prevalence and natural history of adrenal incidentalomas. Eur J Endocrinol 2003;149(4):273–85.
7. Kloos RT, Gross MD, Francis IR, et al. Incidentally discovered adrenal masses. Endocr Rev 1995;16(4):460–84.
8. NIH state-of-the-science statement on management of the clinically inapparent adrenal mass ("incidentaloma"). NIH Consens State Sci Statements 2002;19(2): 1–25.
9. National Comprehensive Cancer Network. NCCN Clinical Practice Guidelines in Oncology: Neuroendocrine Tumors. Version 1.2012. Available at: http://www.nccn.org/professionals/physician_gls/f_guidelines.asp. Accessed May 10, 2012.
10. Deutschbein T, Unger N, Mann K, et al. Diagnosis of secondary adrenal insufficiency in patients with hypothalamic-pituitary disease: comparison between serum and salivary cortisol during the high-dose short synacthen test. Eur J Endocrinol 2009;160:9–16.
11. Bittner JG 4th, Brunt LM. Evaluation and management of adrenal incidentaloma. J Surg Oncol 2012;106(5):557–64.
12. Ilias I, Sahdev A, Reznek RH, et al. The optimal imaging of adrenal tumours: a comparison of different methods. Endocr Relat Cancer 2007;14(3):587–99.
13. Heinz-Peer G, Memarsadeghi M, Niederle B. Imaging of adrenal masses. Curr Opin Urol 2007;17(1):32–8.
14. Pena CS, Boland GW, Hahn PF, et al. Characterization of indeterminate (lipid-poor) adrenal masses: use of washout characteristics at contrast-enhanced CT. Radiology 2000;217(3):798–802.
15. Caoili EM, Korobkin M, Francis IR, et al. Adrenal masses: characterization with combined unenhanced and delayed enhanced CT. Radiology 2002;222(3):629–33.
16. Szolar DH, Korobkin M, Reittner P, et al. Adrenocortical carcinomas and adrenal pheochromocytomas: mass and enhancement loss evaluation at delayed contrast-enhanced CT. Radiology 2005;234(2):479–85.
17. Park BK, Kim CK, Kim B, et al. Comparison of delayed enhanced CT and chemical shift MR for evaluating hyperattenuating incidental adrenal masses. Radiology 2007;243(3):760–5.
18. Sturgeon C, Kebebew E. Laparoscopic adrenalectomy for malignancy. Surg Clin North Am 2004;84(3):755–74.
19. Quayle FJ, Spiltler JA, Pierce RA, et al. Needle biopsy of incidentally discovered adrenal masses is rarely informative and potentially hazardous. Surgery 2007; 142(4):497–502.
20. Fassnacht M, Kenn W, Allolio B. Adrenal tumors: how to establish malignancy? J Endocrinol Invest 2004;27(4):387–99.
21. Schteingart DE, Doherty GM, Gauger PG, et al. Management of patients with adrenal cancer: recommendations of an international consensus conference. Endocr Relat Cancer 2005;12(3):667–80.
22. Allolio B, Fassnacht M. Clinical review: adrenocortical carcinoma: clinical update. J Clin Endocrinol Metab 2006;91(6):2027–37.

23. Eustace D, Han X, Gooding R, et al. Interleukin-6 (IL-6) functions as an autocrine growth factor in cervical carcinomas in vitro. Gynecol Oncol 1993;50(1):15–9.
24. Mornex R, Badet C, Peyrin L. Malignant pheochromocytoma: a series of 14 cases observed between 1996–1990. J Endocrinol Invest 1992;15(9):643–9.
25. Tato A, Orte L, Diz P, et al. Malignant pheochromocytoma, still a therapeutic challenge. Am J Hypertens 1997;10(4 Pt 1):479–81.
26. Schlumberger M, Gicquel C, Lumbroso J, et al. Malignant pheochromocytoma: clinical, biological, histologic and therapeutic data in a series of 20 patients with distant metastases. J Endocrinol Invest 1992;15(9):631–42.
27. Nativ O, Grant CS, Sheps SG, et al. Prognostic profile for patients with pheochromocytoma derived from clinical and pathological factors and DNA ploidy pattern. J Surg Oncol 1992;50(4):258–62.
28. Kaji P, Carrasquillo JA, Linehan WM, et al. The role of 6-[18F]fluorodopamine positron emission tomography in the localization of adrenal pheochromocytoma associated with von Hippel-Lindau syndrome. Eur J Endocrinol 2007;156(4):483–7.
29. Ilias I, Pacak K. Diagnosis and management of tumors of the adrenal medulla. Horm Metab Res 2005;37(12):717–21.
30. Asgreirsson KS, Olafsdottir K, Jonasson JG, et al. The effects of IL-6 on cell adhesion and e-cadherin expression in breast cancer. Cytokine 1998;10(9):720–8.
31. Meyer-Rochow GY, Sidhu SB, Soon PS, et al. Laparoscopic adrenalectomy for pheochromocytoma is safe and effective. Aust N Z J Surg 2007;77(Suppl 1):A25.
32. Kebebew E, Duh QY. Benign and malignant pheochromocytoma: diagnosis, treatment, and follow-up. Surg Oncol Clin North Am 1998;7(4):765–89.
33. Mahoney EM, Harrison JH. Malignant pheochromocytoma: clinical course and treatment. J Urol 1977;118(2):225–9.
34. Tanaka S, Ito T, Tomoda J, et al. Malignant pheochromocytoma with hepatic metastasis diagnosed 20 years after resection of the primary adrenal lesion. Intern Med 1993;32(10):789–94.
35. Dackiw AP, Lee JE, Gagel RF, et al. Adrenal cortical carcinoma. World J Surg 2001;25(7):914–26.
36. Solcia E, Rindi G, Paolotti D, et al. Clinicopathological profile as a basis for classification of the endocrine tumours of the gastroenteropancreatic tract. Ann Oncol 1999;10(Suppl 2):S9–15.
37. Crucitti F, Bellantone R, Ferrante A, et al. The Italian Registry for Adrenal Cortical Carcinoma: analysis of a multiinstitutional series of 129 patients. The ACC Italian Registry Study Group. Surgery 1996;119(2):161–70.
38. Wooten MD, King DK. Adrenal cortical carcinoma. Epidemiology and treatment with mitotane and a review of the literature. Cancer 1993;72(11):3145–55.
39. Marx S, Spiegal AM, Skarulis MC, et al. Multiple endocrine neoplasia type 1: clinical and genetic topics. Ann Intern Med 1998;129(6):484–94.
40. Kock CA, Pacak K, Chrousos GP. The molecular pathogenesis of hereditary and sporadic adrenocortical and adrenomedullary tumors. J Clin Endocrinol Metab 2002;87(12):5367–84.
41. Lynch HT, Radford B, Lynch J. SBLA syndrome revisited. Oncology 1990;47(1):75–9.
42. Soon PS, McDonald KL, Robinson BG, et al. Molecular markers and the pathogenesis of adrenocortical cancer. Oncologist 2008;13(5):548–61.
43. Brandi ML, Gagel RF, Angeli A, et al. Guidelines for diagnosis and therapy of MEN type 1 and type 2. J Clin Endocrinol Metab 2001;86(12):5658–71.
44. Ohgaki H, Kleihues P, Heitz PU. p53 mutations in sporadic adrenocortical tumors. Int J Cancer 1993;54(3):408–10.

45. Reincke M, Karl M, Travis WH, et al. p53 mutations in human adrenocortical neoplasms: immunohistochemical and molecular studies. J Clin Endocrinol Metab 1994;78(3):790–4.
46. Gicquel C, Bertagna X, Schneid H, et al. Rearrangements at the 11p15 locus and overexpression of insulin-like growth factor-II gene in sporadic adrenocortical tumors. J Clin Endocrinol Metab 1994;78(6):1444–53.
47. Gicquel C, Raffin-Sanson ML, Gaston V, et al. Structural and functional abnormalities at 11p15 are associated with the malignant phenotype in sporadic adrenocortical tumors: study on a series of 82 tumors. J Clin Endocrinol Metab 1997; 82(8):2559–65.
48. Ng L, Libertino JM. Adrenocortical carcinoma: diagnosis, evaluation and treatment. J Urol 2003;169(1):5–11.
49. Bertagna C, Orth DN. Clinical and laboratory findings and results of therapy in 58 patients with adrenocortical tumors admitted to a single medical center (1951 to 1978). Am J Med 1981;71(5):855–75.
50. Luton JP, Cerdas S, Billaud L, et al. Clinical features of adrenocortical carcinoma, prognostic factors, and the effect of mitotane therapy. N Engl J Med 1990; 322(17):1195–201.
51. Latronico AC, Chrousos GP. Extensive personal experience: adrenocortical tumors. J Clin Endocrinol Metab 1997;82(5):1317–24.
52. Kasperlik-Zaluska AA, Migdalska BM, Zgliczynski S, et al. Adrenocortical carcinoma. A clinical study and treatment results of 52 patients. Cancer 1995; 75(10):2587–91.
53. Arnold DT, Reed JB, Burt K. Evaluation and management of the incidental adrenal mass. Proc (Bayl Univ Med Cent) 2003;16(1):7–12.
54. Barzon L, Zucchetta P, Boscaro M, et al. Scintigraphic patterns of adrenocortical carcinomas: morpho-functional correlates. Eur J Endocrinol 2001;145(6): 743–8.
55. Favia G, Lumachi F, D'Amico DF. Adrenocortical carcinoma: is prognosis different in nonfunctioning tumors? Results of surgical treatment in 31 patients. World J Surg 2001;25(6):735–8.
56. Kasperlik-Zaluska AA, Migdalska B, Makowska A. Incidentally found adrenocortical carcinoma. A study of 21 patients. Eur J Cancer 1998;34(11):1721–4.
57. Vassilopoulou-Sellin R, Schultz PN. Adrenocortical carcinoma. Clinical outcome at the end of the 20th century. Cancer 2001;92(5):1113–21.
58. Wajchenberg BL, Albergaria Pereira MA, Medonca BB, et al. Adrenocortical carcinoma: clinical and laboratory observations. Cancer 2000;88(4):711–36.
59. Pommier RF, Brennan MF. An eleven-year experience with adrenocortical carcinoma. Surgery 1992;112(6):963–70 [discussion: 970–1].
60. Porpiglia F, Miller BS, Manfredi M, et al. A debate on laparoscopic versus open adrenalectomy for adrenocortical carcinoma. Horm Cancer 2011;2(6):372–7.
61. Ushiyama T, Suzuki K, Kageyama S, et al. A case of Cushing's syndrome due to adrenocortical carcinoma with recurrence 19 months after laparoscopic adrenalectomy. J Urol 1997;157(6):2239.
62. Hofle G, Gasser RW, Lhotta K, et al. Adrenocortical carcinoma evolving after diagnosis of preclinical Cushing's syndrome in an adrenal incidentaloma. A case report. Horm Res 1998;50(4):237–42.
63. Hamoir E, Meurisse M, Defechereux T. Is laparoscopic resection of malignant corticoadrenaloma feasible? Case report of early, diffuse and massive peritoneal recurrence after attempted laparoscopic resection. Ann Chir 1998;52(4): 364–8.

64. Deckers S, Derdelinckx L, Col V, et al. Peritoneal carcinomatosis following laparoscopic resection of an adrenocortical tumor causing primary hyperaldosteronism. Horm Res 1999;52(2):97–100.
65. Foxius A, Ramboux A, Lefebvre Y, et al. Hazards of laparoscopic adrenalectomy for Conn's adenoma. When enthusiasm turns to tragedy. Surg Endosc 1999; 13(7):715–7.
66. McCauley LR, Nguyen MM. Laparoscopic radical adrenalectomy for cancer: long-term outcomes. Curr Opin Urol 2008;18(2):134–8.
67. Gonzalez RJ, Shapiro S, Sarlis N, et al. Laparoscopic resection of adrenal cortical carcinoma: a cautionary note. Surgery 2005;138(6):1078–85 [discussion: 1085–6].
68. Porpiglia F, Fiori C, Tarabuzzi R, et al. Is laparoscopic adrenalectomy feasible for adrenocortical carcinoma or metastasis? BJU Int 2004;94(7):1026–9.
69. Porpiglia F, Fiori C, Daffara F, et al. Retrospective evaluation of the outcome of open versus laparoscopic adrenalectomy for stage I and II adrenocortical cancer. Eur Urol 2010;57(5):873–8.
70. Brix D, Allolio B, Fenske W, et al. Laparoscopic versus open adrenalectomy for adrenocortical carcinoma: surgical and oncologic outcome in 152 patients. Eur Urol 2010;58(4):609–15.
71. Leboulleux S, Deanderis D, Al Ghuzian A, et al. Adrenocortical carcinoma: is the surgical approach a risk factor of peritoneal carcinomatosis? Eur J Endocrinol 2010;162(6):1147–53.
72. Miller BS, Ammori JB, Gauger PG, et al. Laparoscopic resection is inappropriate in patients with known or suspected adrenocortical carcinoma. World J Surg 2010;34(6):1380–5.
73. Saunders BD, Doherty GM. Laparoscopic adrenalectomy for malignant disease. Lancet Oncol 2004;5:718–26.
74. Shen WT, Sturgeon C, Duh QY. From incidentaloma to adrenocortical carcinoma: the surgical management of adrenal tumors. J Surg Oncol 2005;89:186–92.
75. Heniford BT, Iannitti DA, Hale J, et al. The role of intraoperative ultrasonography during laparoscopic adrenalectomy. Surgery 1997;122(6):1068–73.
76. Assalia A, Gagner M. Laparoscopic adrenalectomy. Br J Surg 2004;91(10): 1259–74.
77. Henry JF, Sebag F, Iacobone M, et al. Lessons learned from 274 laparoscopic adrenalectomies. Ann Chir 2002;127(7):512–9.
78. Curet MJ. Port site metastases. Am J Surg 2004;187(6):705–12.
79. Gonzalez R, Smith CD, McClusky DA 3rd, et al. Laparoscopic approach reduces likelihood of perioperative complications in patients undergoing adrenalectomy. Am Surg 2004;70(8):668–74.
80. Suzuki K, Ushiyama T, Mugiya S, et al. Hazards of laparoscopic adrenalectomy in patients with adrenal malignancy. J Urol 1997;158(6):2227.
81. Abecassis M, McLoughlin MJ, Langer B, et al. Serendipitous adrenal masses: prevalence, significance, and management. Am J Surg 1985;149(6):783–8.
82. Belldegrun A, Hussain S, Seltzer SE, et al. Incidentally discovered mass of the adrenal gland. Surg Gynecol Obstet 1986;163(3):203–8.
83. Caplan RH, Strutt PJ, Wickus GG. Subclinical hormone secretion by incidentally discovered adrenal masses. Arch Surg 1994;129(3):291–6.
84. Guerrieri M, De Sanctis A, Crosta F, et al. Adrenal incidentaloma: surgical update. J Endocrinol Invest 2007;30(3):200–4.
85. Ayabe H, Tsuji H, Hara D, et al. Surgical management of adrenal metastasis from bronchogenic carcinoma. J Surg Oncol 1995;58(3):149–54.

86. Kim SH, Brennan MF, Russo P, et al. The role of surgery in the treatment of clinically isolated adrenal metastasis. Cancer 1998;82(2):389–94.
87. Sarela AI, Murphy I, Coit DG, et al. Metastasis to the adrenal gland: the emerging role of laparoscopic surgery. Ann Surg Oncol 2003;10:1191–6.
88. Weyhe D, Belyaev O, Skawran S, et al. A case of port-site recurrence after laparoscopic adrenalectomy for solitary adrenal metastasis. Surg Laparosc Endosc Percutan Tech 2007;17(3):218–20.
89. Saraiva P, Rodrigues H, Rodrigues P. Port site recurrence after laparoscopic adrenalectomy for metastatic melanoma. Int Braz J Urol 2003;29(6):520–1.
90. Rassweiler J, Tsivian A, Kumar AV, et al. Oncological safety of laparoscopic surgery for urological malignancy: experience with more than 1,000 operations. J Urol 2003;169(6):2072–5.
91. Chen B, Zhou M, Cappelli MC, et al. Port site, retroperitoneal and intra-abdominal recurrence after laparoscopic adrenalectomy for apparently isolated metastasis. J Urol 2002;168(6):2528–9.
92. Adler JT, Mack E, Chen H. Equal oncologic results for laparoscopic and open resection of adrenal metastases. J Surg Res 2007;140(2):159–64.
93. Strong VE, D'Angelica M, Tang L, et al. Laparoscopic adrenalectomy for isolated adrenal metastasis. Ann Surg Oncol 2007;14(12):3392–400.
94. Valeri A, Borrelli A, Presenti L, et al. Adrenal masses in neoplastic patients: the role of laparoscopic procedure. Surg Endosc 2001;15(1):90–3.
95. Muth A, Persson F, Jansson S, et al. Prognostic factors for survival after adrenal metastasis. Eur J Surg Oncol 2010;36(7):699–704.
96. Sancho JJ, Triponez F, Montet X, et al. Surgical management of adrenal metastases. Langenbecks Arch Surg 2012;397(2):179–94.

Laparoscopic Prostatectomy for Prostate Cancer
Continued Role in Urology

Gurdarshan S. Sandhu, MD, Kenneth G. Nepple, MD,
Youssef S. Tanagho, MD, MPH, Gerald L. Andriole, MD*

KEYWORDS

- Laparoscopic prostatectomy • Prostatectomy • Prostate neoplasms
- Prostate cancer • Outcomes

KEY POINTS

- Laparoscopic prostatectomy has perioperative outcomes that are similar to open and robotic-assisted laparoscopic approaches.
- Laparoscopic prostatectomy yields short- and intermediate-term oncologic outcomes that are similar to open radical retropubic prostatectomy.
- Laparoscopic prostatectomy has functional outcomes (urinary continence and potency) that are similar to open radical retropubic prostatectomy.
- Laparoscopic prostatectomy is a more cost-effective minimally invasive approach than a robotic-assisted procedure and can approximate cost equivalence to an open approach.

Prostate cancer is the most common noncutaneous malignancy in men, accounting for 240 890 new cases in 2011.[1] The introduction of serum prostate-specific antigen (PSA) as a screening test in the 1980s[2] aided the detection of prostate cancer[3] and contributed to the increased incidence. Additionally, with the widespread adoption of PSA screening as a public health initiative in the United States, a well-documented stage migration has been noted with a marked increase in the frequency of diagnosis of asymptomatic, clinically localized disease.[4,5] A population-based analysis has revealed that greater than 90% of newly diagnosed men have localized disease (T1 or T2) that does not extend beyond the capsule of the prostate or involve the seminal vesicles.[4]

Disclosures: Gerald L. Andriole serves as medical director for Viking Systems.
Division of Urologic Surgery, Washington University School of Medicine, Campus Box 8242, 4960 Children's Place, St Louis, MO 63110, USA
* Corresponding author.
E-mail address: andrioleg@wustl.edu

Surg Oncol Clin N Am 22 (2013) 125–141
http://dx.doi.org/10.1016/j.soc.2012.08.001
1055-3207/13/$ – see front matter © 2013 Elsevier Inc. All rights reserved.

There are several treatment options for patients with localized disease, including active surveillance, brachytherapy, radiation therapy, focal therapy (ie, cryosurgery), or surgery. Of these options, level I evidence supporting a survival benefit compared with no treatment is unique to surgery,[6] whereas the other treatments have not been adequately studied in a randomized fashion.

Currently, there are several surgical approaches to radical prostatectomy, including perineal prostatectomy, open radical retropubic prostatectomy, laparoscopic prostatectomy, and robotic-assisted laparoscopic prostatectomy (RALP). In practice, the choice of surgical approach is primarily based on surgeon and patient preference. This review aims to explore the role of laparoscopic prostatectomy in the management of prostate cancer.

HISTORY OF LAPAROSCOPIC PROSTATECTOMY

Hugh Hampton Young[7] performed the first open prostatectomy for prostate cancer via a perineal incision in 1905. This achievement was followed by the first description of the traditional radical retropubic prostatectomy by Millin in 1947. Several anatomic studies in the 1970s and 1980s allowed for a better appreciation of periprostatic anatomy and consequent reduction in operative morbidity.[8–10] In an attempt to further decrease operative morbidity and improve postoperative convalescence, minimally invasive techniques were applied to prostatectomy.

Shuessler and colleagues[11] described the initial series of laparoscopic prostatectomy in 1997, reporting on the short-term outcomes of 9 patients. The investigators found that the procedure was feasible, but lengthy operative times (average of 9.3 hours) and postoperative stay (average of 7.3 days) precluded any distinct advantage over open surgery. As a result of these findings and the technical difficulty of a laparoscopic approach, the urologic community did not immediately adopt the procedure.

Interest in laparoscopic prostatectomy was rekindled following the dissemination of the experience from 2 centers in France.[12–14] Using a reproducible stepwise approach, the operative times in these series were more acceptable (4–5 hours) as were the positive margin rates (15%–28%) and functional outcomes. This technique was subsequently adopted by several centers with surgeons who had the necessary laparoscopic skills.

It is noteworthy that laparoscopic prostatectomy remains a procedure with a challenging learning curve. The number of cases required to become proficient generally ranges from 200 to 700 in the published literature.[15–22] The learning curve varies for different stages of the procedure,[15,18] with more challenging steps, such as completion of the vesicourethral anastomosis or optimization of nerve sparing, requiring a higher case volume for proficiency. Attempts to decrease the length of the learning curve have included a rigorous mentored approach[23] as well as completion of a fellowship that encompasses minimally invasive techniques.[16] Others have also found that extensive open prostatectomy experience may not shorten the learning curve for laparoscopic prostatectomy; instead, the curve may be more abbreviated with prior laparoscopic experience.[17,22]

INDICATIONS AND CONTRAINDICATIONS

Laparoscopic prostatectomy has identical indications to that of open prostatectomy, primarily being a treatment option offered to patients with organ-confined, nonmetastatic disease. Preliminary results regarding the safety and feasibility of salvage laparoscopic prostatectomy have also been described in several small, single-institution series following radiation therapy or high-intensity focused ultrasound.[24–29] Because prior treatment can obliterate natural tissue planes and result in periprostatic fibrosis with an attendant increase in potential complications, such as rectal injury, it is advisable that such salvage cases be avoided in a surgeon's early experience with laparoscopic prostatectomy.

Absolute contraindications to laparoscopic prostatectomy include the conventional contraindications to standard laparoscopy, such as cardiopulmonary insufficiency or coagulopathy. Although additional factors, such as prior abdominal surgery[30–32] and morbid obesity,[33,34] are not necessarily contraindications to laparoscopic prostatectomy, they remain important preoperative considerations insofar as they can increase the difficulty of the surgery and increase the risk of open conversion early in a surgeon's learning curve.[35] Larger prostate glands (>70 g) can also result in increased operative times, blood loss, and postoperative stay.[36,37]

INSTRUMENTATION AND APPROACH

The instrumentation (**Table 1**) required to perform laparoscopic prostatectomy depends to some extent on the surgical approach (transperitoneal vs extraperitoneal) as well as surgeon preference.

Extraperitoneal versus Transperitoneal Approach

The extraperitoneal approach offers several potential intraoperative and postoperative advantages and is currently preferred at the authors' institution. This approach allows patients to remain supine and avoid some complications related to the steep Trendelenburg positioning required with a transperitoneal approach.[38–41] Intraoperatively, avoiding peritoneotomy allows the peritoneum to contain the bowels and prevents them from obscuring the view of the surgical field. Similarly, this may serve to protect the bowels from inadvertent injury. The extraperitoneal approach also avoids some of the difficulty associated with bowel adhesions from prior surgery, which can complicate a transperitoneal approach. Postoperatively, if a urine leak from the vesicourethral anastomosis should develop, it remains confined to the extraperitoneal space

Table 1
Suggested instruments for laparoscopic prostatectomy

5-mm trocars (3) 12-mm trocars (3)	Trocar-mounted balloon-dilator device
0° and 30° laparoscope lens, camera holder	Viking 3DHD Vision System (Viking Systems, Westborough, Massachusetts)
Suction-irrigation device 10 mm	Monopolar scissors
Bipolar forceps: fine and broad	PEER retractor (JARIT Surgical Instruments Inc, Hawthorne, New York) and Endoholder (Codman, Raynham, Massachusetts)
Laparoscopic needle drivers (2)	Sutures: 0 polyglactin suture on a CT-1 needle for dorsal venous complex; 2-0 polyglactin suture on an SH needle for bladder neck reconstruction; double-arm 2-0 poliglecaprone on an SH needle for vesicourethral anastomosis
Locking, toothed prostate clamp	Hem-o-Lok clips (Teleflex Medical, Research Triangle Park, North Carolina) and Lapra-Ty suture clips (Ethicon Endosurgery, Cincinnati, Ohio)
24F (initial) and 18F (final) urethral catheters	

and does not cause peritonitis. Alternatively, if a lymphocele occurs after the extraperitoneal approach, it may be more apt to be symptomatic because the lymphatic fluid is not reabsorbed by contact with the bowel and peritoneal membrane. Although these advantages may come at a potential cost of a decreased operative working space as compared with a transperitoneal approach, a laparoscopic extraperitoneal prostatectomy can still be safely performed in obese patients and/or those with large prostates.[42]

Several retrospective nonrandomized series have compared these approaches[43–48] and have generally found that operative time and time to return to continence are shorter with the extraperitoneal approach,[43,45,46] although these measures are surgeon dependent. Measures of blood loss or transfusion rates,[43,44,46,48] positive surgical margins (PSM),[43–45,47,48] and long-term continence have been similar between the two approaches. In practice, completion of the procedure is feasible and safe with both approaches, and the decision on which approach to use is largely dictated by surgeon preference and prior experience.

TECHNIQUE

The steps for performing laparoscopic prostatectomy vary slightly between the transperitoneal and extraperitoneal approaches. For the purposes of this review, the operative steps for an extraperitoneal approach are described. Although a formal description of the operative approach is beyond the scope of this review, the procedure can be divided into several reproducible steps.

The patient is positioned supine on the operating table. A 1.5-cm midline incision (later used as the extraction incision) is made just caudal to the umbilicus. The incision is deepened through the midline fascia, and the extraperitoneal space is developed with blunt finger dissection, taking care to not enter a plane between the deep inferior epigastric arteries and the undersurface of the rectus muscles. After a sufficient space has been obtained, a 6-trocar technique is used, including two 12-mm trocars and four 5-mm trocars. Under digital guidance, a 5-mm trocar is placed to the left of the incision in the midclavicular line and a 12-mm port is similarly placed to the right. A balloon trocar is placed through the midline incision and insufflation is performed. Two 5-mm trocars are placed near the anterior superior iliac spines bilaterally, and one is placed near the midline between the pubic symphysis and the umbilicus under direct vision (**Fig. 1**). The surgeon stands on the left side of the patient and the Endoholder (Codman, Raynham, Massachusetts) is anchored to the operating table, allowing for fixed retraction through the left lower quadrant 5-mm trocar and facilitating the remainder of the procedure.[49] Similarly, a camera holder is also fixed to the head end of the operating table to allow for hands-free support of the camera. Both the Endoholder and camera holder free the hands of the surgical assistant and surgeon and expedite the procedure. Additionally, the authors have adopted the use of the Viking 3DHD Vision System (Viking Systems, Westborough, Massachusetts) for this procedure because it facilitates intraoperative vision and can decrease the learning curve of complex laparoscopic procedures.[50]

After establishing insufflation ($\sim$15 mm Hg), bilateral pelvic lymph node dissections are performed. All node-bearing tissue is removed from the obturator fossa and alongside the internal and external iliac arteries and veins bilaterally. Lymphatic attachments are cauterized with bipolar energy and then divided. Care is taken to preserve the obturator nerve and vessels during this dissection. More extensive node dissections are performed for men with intermediate- and high-risk tumors.[51] The endopelvic fascia is then incised sharply and the puboprostatic ligaments are

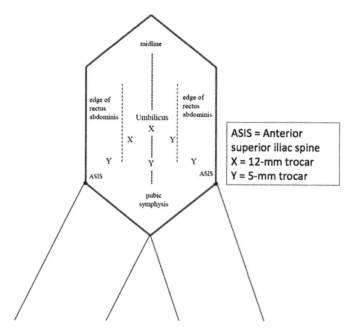

Fig. 1. Port placement for laparoscopic prostatectomy.

divided, thereby allowing accurate identification of the dorsal venous complex (DVC). The DVC is then suture ligated with a 0-polyglactin suture on a CT-1 needle. The use of a pledget and a Lapra-Ty suture clip (Ethicon Endosurgery, Cincinnati, Ohio) facilitate this because knot tying beneath the pubic symphysis can be time consuming.

The bladder neck is then identified by movement of the Foley catheter and transected widely, distal to the ureteral orifices. Indigo carmine is given earlier in the procedure to help identify the ureteral orifices and verify that iatrogenic injury has not occurred. After division of the posterior bladder neck, the vasa deferentia and seminal vesicles are individually identified, completely mobilized, and divided. Anterior traction on the prostate through the midline 5-mm trocar site and posterior-cranial retraction of the bladder using the left lower quadrant port allows for easier dissection of the seminal vesicles and development of the plane between the prostate and rectum. The prostatic pedicles are controlled with a series of Hem-o-Lok clips (Teleflex Medical, Research Triangle Park, North Carolina) and divided sharply, avoiding cautery given the proximity of the neurovascular bundles. For men with low-risk cancers, the neurovascular bundles are gently mobilized off of the prostate laterally after a high release of levator fascia surrounding the prostate, thereby preserving a veil of tissue (veil of Aphrodite) containing nerves important for erectile function.[52] Classic nerve-sparing or non–nerve-sparing techniques are performed for men with more advanced tumors if the dissection is difficult because of the adherence of the neurovascular bundles to the prostate.

The apical dissection is performed next, which begins with transection of the previously ligated DVC, then the urethra (just distal to the apex of the prostate) and rectourethral muscle. The specimen is then entrapped within a laparoscopic entrapment sac and removed by lengthening the midline fasciotomy. The surgeon can inspect the prostate to determine the adequacy of the dissection while the assistant closes the fasciotomy and reestablishes pelvic insufflation. The wide bladder neck is then reconstructed in a tennis racquet fashion using a 2-0 polyglactin suture on an SH needle, so that the opening in the bladder better approximates the urethral lumen. Finally, the vesicourethral anastomosis is performed using a running double-arm 2-0 polyglyconate suture in the van Velthoven method[53] and secured with Lapra-Ty clips (Ethicon EndoSurgery, Cincinnati, Ohio).

PERIOPERATIVE OUTCOMES

There are no randomized studies comparing open laparoscopic and robotic-assisted approaches to prostatectomy. Most of the published reports are retrospective single-center case series, which suggest comparable outcomes across these surgical approaches (**Table 2**). However, comparisons between published series are obscured by differences in patient populations, surgeon experience, and measures of outcome.

Operative Time

Operative times for laparoscopic prostatectomy by experienced practitioners are generally comparable with open radical retropubic prostatectomy. These times have been shown to consistently decrease with increasing surgical experience across the published literature. At centers of excellence, the operative time has been reported to be in the range of 2.5 to 4.0 hours depending on the experience of the operating surgeon (see **Table 2**).

Intraoperative Blood Loss

A laparoscopic approach offers the benefit of a tamponading effect from the pneumo-peritoneum, which is especially relevant when performing a prostatectomy because most of the intraoperative blood loss is related to bleeding from venous sinuses, such as the dorsal venous complex. Additionally, the improved visualization with laparoscopy allows for potentially more meticulous dissection and control of bleeding vessels. In most series, the intraoperative blood loss is 400 mL or less (see **Table 2**) and has been generally found to be less than that seen with open radical retropubic prostatectomy in most comparative studies.[54–61] A more meaningful parameter may be the transfusion rate, which ranges from 0% to 11% in the published literature (see **Table 2**) and has also been shown to be significantly less than that seen with open radical prostatectomy in many series.[57–62]

Hospital Stay

A significant difference in hospital stay between a laparoscopic and open prostatec-tomy has become more difficult to demonstrate because the length of stay has decreased dramatically with open surgery (perhaps in response to shorter initial hospital stays with laparoscopic surgery), with some high-volume centers reporting postoperative stays of 1 to 2 days following open prostatectomy.[63] However, a recent population-based analysis did find that laparoscopic prostatectomy was associated with a statistically significant decrease in length of stay (based on data from 2008).[64] Currently, at the authors' center (and many others), most patients are routinely discharged on postoperative day 1, with some patients discharged on the same day of surgery.

ONCOLOGIC OUTCOMES

Postoperative oncologic control can be evaluated using surrogate measures, such as the absence of a PSM or freedom from biochemical recurrence (BCR) (PSA recur-rence) in series in which the follow-up is not mature enough to yield more conventional

Table 2
Perioperative outcomes of radical prostatectomy performed in selected series

Reference	Approach	No	Mean Operative Time	Mean EBL (mL)	Transfusion (%)	Mean LOS (d)	Complications (%)	PSM
Lein et al[94]	TLRP	1000	266	—	2.2	—	11.8	pT2 14.9 / pT3 54.5 / pT4 100
Rassweiler et al[79]	TLRP: early group	219	288	1100	30.1	12.0	19.6	21.0
	TLRP: late group	219	218	800	9.6	11.0	10.5	23.7
Eden et al[95]	TLRP	100	245	313	3.0	3.8	8.0	16.0
Guillonneau et al[81]	TLRP	550	200	380	5.3	5.8	10.0	15.0
Rozet et al[82]	ELRP	600	173	380	1.2	6.3	11.5	17.7
Ferguson et al[96]	ELRP	420	–	350	1.4	1.27	—	pT2 19.1 / pT3 44.3 / pT4 100
Cohen et al[97]	ELRP	172	170	176	0	1.67	9.9	14.5
Goeman et al[98]	ELRP	550	188	390	4.7	4.6	10.9	pT2 17.9 / pT3 44.8 / pT4 71.4
Stolzenburg et al[83]	ELRP	700	151	220	0.9	—	2.4	pT2 10.8 / pT3 31.2
German Group[72]	TLRP (n = 3935) ELRP (n = 1889)	5824	196	—	4.1	—	8.9	pT2 10.6 / pT3a 32.0 / pT3b 56.0
Stolzenburg et al[99]	ELRP	2000	156	—	0.6	9.0	Intraoperative: 0.5 / Early postoperative: 8.6 / Late postoperative: 0.3	pT2 9.7 / pT3 34.4
Rassweiler et al[79]	ORP	219	196	1550	55.7	16.0	35.6	28.7
Zincke et al[100]	ORP	3170	—	600–1030	5.0–31.0	—	—	24.0
Lepor et al[101]	ORP	1000	—	819	9.7	2.3	7.0	19.9

Abbreviations: EBL, estimated blood loss; ELRP, extraperitoneal laparoscopic radical prostatectomy; LOS, length of stay; ORP, open radical retropubic prostatectomy; TLRP, transperitoneal laparoscopic radical prostatectomy.

outcomes, such as cancer-specific and overall survival. Many laparoscopic prostatectomy series have limited follow-up because the procedure began to gain wider use
only after the year 2000.

PSM Rate

The overall PSM rate for laparoscopic prostatectomy ranges from 11% to 31%
(see **Table 2; Table 3**). The rate of PSM is dependent on surgeon experience, disease
characteristics of the patient cohort, and pathologic processing of the specimen. In
comparative studies, there is only one randomized trial[58] and one prospective study.[56]
In the randomized trial, which included a single surgeon and 120 patients, no difference was found in PSM rates between the open and laparoscopic approaches for
the overall cohort (26% vs 22%, $P = .28$), those with organ-confined disease, and

Table 3
Oncologic outcomes of radical prostatectomy performed in selected series

Reference	Approach	No	Global	T2	T3a	T3b	5 y	10 y
			Positive Margins (%)				**Freedom From BCR (%)**	
Curto et al[84]	LRP	413	30.7	T2a: 7.4 T2b: 21.0 T2c: 24.0	43.0	46.0	—	—
German Group[72]	LRP	5824	—	10.6	32.0	56.0	pT2: 91.4 pT3: 82.5	—
Rassweiler et al[69]	LRP	500	19.0	7.4	25.2	42.0	73.1	—
Rozet et al[82]	LRP	600	17.7	14.6	25.6	—	95.0 (1 y)	—
Guillonneau et al[102]	LRP	1000	19.2	T2a: 6.9 T2b: 18.6	30.0	34.0	90.5 (3 y)	—
Pavlovich et al[103]	LRP	508	—	8.2	pT3: 39.3	—	pT2: 98.2 (3 y) pT3: 78.7 (3 y)	—
Tai et al[70]	LRP	218	—	14.6	pT3: 48.6	—	74.5	—
Paul et al[71]	LRP	1115	—	16.1	pT3: 34.6	—	Overall: 83 pT2: 93.4 pT3a: 74.5 pT3b: 55.0	—
Comparative studies between RRP and LRP								
Guazzoni et al[58]	RRP	60	21.6	18.2	31.2	—	—	—
	LRP	60	26.0	24.4	33.0			
Touijer et al[61]	RRP	818	11.0	—	—	—	—	—
	LRP	612	11.0					
Roumeguere et al[56]	RRP	77	40.2	7.3	—	—	—	—
	LRP	85	25.8	7.8				
Rassweiler et al[79]	RRP	219	28.7	17.0	30.6	52.4	82.6	—
	LRP (EG)	219	21.0	11.9	17.3	54.3	86.8 (30 mo)	
	LRP (LG)	219	23.7	18.0	38.8	54.5		
Jurczok et al[59]	RRP	240	19.6	12.6	—	—	—	—
	LRP	163	16.6	9.8				
Anastadiasis et al[62]	RRP	70	28.6	—	—	—	—	—
	LRP	230	26.5					

Abbreviations: EG, early group; LG, late group; LRP, laparoscopic radical prostatectomy; RRP, open
retropubic radical prostatectomy.

those with extraprostatic extension of disease.[58] Similarly, no differences were found in the prospective trial when the PSM rates were stratified by pathologic stage.[56] A systematic review of the literature also found no difference in PSM rates between open and laparoscopic approaches.[65] Similarly, no difference in PSM rates has been observed in comparative studies between laparoscopic and robotic-assisted approaches.[65–68]

Freedom from BCR

The published literature reporting on BCR following laparoscopic prostatectomy largely consists of single-surgeon or institution series (see **Table 3**). Furthermore, the reported outcomes are limited to short and intermediate follow-up, given the recent adoption of this surgical approach. Moreover, BCR has been defined in multiple different ways (eg, PSA >0.1, PSA >0.20, 2 increases of PSA more than PSA >0.20, initiation of additional treatment).

The 5-year freedom from BCR ranges from 73% to 83%,[69–71] with the German laparoscopic working group having reported 5-year BCR freedom of 91.4% for organ-confined disease and 82.5% in the presence of extraprostatic extension.[72] These outcomes are similar to those of large open prostatectomy series (5-year freedom from BCR 70%–92%).[73–76]

FUNCTIONAL OUTCOMES

It remains somewhat difficult to interpret reported functional outcomes after laparoscopic prostatectomy because there is a lack of uniformity in defining and assessing outcomes, such as urinary continence and erectile function, which likely contributes to some of the observed differences between published studies.

Urinary Continence

There are few published series using validated questionnaires[77,78] to assess postoperative urinary continence after prostatectomy. Continence is typically qualified by the number of daily protective pads worn by patients, with most published literature defining continence as the use of 0 or 1 pads over a 24-hour period.

Urinary continence at 12 months postoperatively ranges from 48% to 95% in the major published series (**Table 4**). Three studies comparing open and laparoscopic prostatectomy found no difference in urinary continence postoperatively between approaches.[56,62,79] However, one study comparing outcomes between the same approaches among surgeons who were beyond the learning curve found that a laparoscopic approach was associated with decreased continence postoperatively (hazard ratio 0.56, 95% confidence interval 0.44–0.70).[61] Based on a cumulative analysis and a systematic review of the literature, the postoperative urinary continence rate was found to be similar between the open and laparoscopic approaches[65] and, at 12 months (based on a 0-pad definition), was reported to be 81% for open radical prostatectomy and 87% for laparoscopic radical prostatectomy.[80] No difference in urinary continence was seen between laparoscopic and robotic-assisted approaches at 6 months postoperatively in a single retrospective study.[66]

Potency

The potency rate, defined as the ability to have intercourse with or without the use of additional medication, at 12 months following laparoscopic prostatectomy ranges from 52% to 78% (see **Table 4**).[79,81–89] In 3 comparative studies between laparoscopic and open prostatectomy, no difference was seen favoring either approach in

Table 4
Functional outcomes of radical prostatectomy performed in selected series

Reference	Approach	Continence				Potency			
		No	Defn	12 mo (%)	24 mo (%)	No	Defn	12 mo (%)	24 mo (%)
Salomon et al[85]	LRP	100	0 pad	90.0	—	77	Intercourse	59	—
Link et al[87]	LRP	122	0–1 pad	93.0	—	122	Intercourse	78	—
Turk et al[89]	LRP	125	0–1 pad	92.0 (9 mo)	—	44	Intercourse	59 (9 mo)	—
Hoznek et al[86]	LRP	134	0 pad	86.2	—	134	Erection	56	—
Curto et al[84]	LRP	202	0 pad	95.0	—	137	Intercourse	59	—
Guilloneau et al[81]	LRP	341	0 pad	82.0	—	41	Intercourse	66	—
Stolzenburg et al[83]	LRP	420	0 pad	92.0	—	83	Intercourse	47 (6 mo)	—
Rassweiler et al[88]	LRP	500	0 pad	83.0	—	41	Intercourse	67	—
Rozet et al[82]	LRP	599	0 pad	84.0	—	599	Intercourse	43 (6 mo)	—
German Group[72]	LRP	5824	0 pad	85.0	—	5824	Intercourse	52	—
Comparative studies between LRP and RRP									
Roumeguere et al[56]	RRP	77	0 pad	83.9	—	77	Intercourse	55	—
	LRP	85	0 pad	80.7	—	85	Intercourse	65	—
Anastisiadis et al[62]	RRP	70	0 pad	66.7	—	70	Intercourse	46	—
	LRP	230	0 pad	71.6	—	230	Intercourse	53	—
Touijer et al[61]	RRP	222	0 pad	75.0	82	222	Intercourse	—	58.5
	LRP	193	0 pad	48.0	62	193	Intercourse	—	56.0
Rassweiler et al[79]	RRP	219	0 pad	89.9	—	—	—	—	—
	LRP	219	0 pad	90.0	—	—	—	—	—
	LRP	219	0 pad	91.7	—	—	—	—	—

Abbreviations: Defn, definition; LRP, laparoscopic radical prostatectomy; RRP, open retropubic radical prostatectomy.

terms of postoperative erectile function.[56,61,62] Similarly, no difference was seen between laparoscopic radical prostatectomy and RALP in terms of erectile function in a retrospective study.[66]

COST COMPARISONS

An additional important consideration with the adoption of a new surgical approach is the cost difference compared with the previous accepted standard. Several series have compared the costs of laparoscopic prostatectomy with the more traditional approach of open radical retropubic prostatectomy.[90–93] The additive cost of a laparoscopic prostatectomy compared with an open approach ranges from $487 to $1507.[91–93] Most of the increased costs attributed to the laparoscopic procedure are related to surgical supply costs (differences ranging from $533–$1057) and operating room costs (differences ranging from $460–$842).[91–93] It has been suggested that the shorter hospital stay can offset the additive operating room costs.[91]

Link and colleagues[90] used a model to evaluate the additional cost of laparoscopic prostatectomy and found that cost equivalence could only be achieved if reusable instruments and trocars were used, the operative time was shorter than 3.4 hours, and patients were discharged on postoperative day 2. In this model, cost parity could not be achieved by simply shortening hospital stay unless laparoscopic prostatectomy was to be done as an outpatient procedure.

Provided operative times and the use of reusable instruments are optimized, the laparoscopic procedure can, therefore, approach the open approach in terms of cost-effectiveness while offering a much cheaper alternative to the robotic-assisted laparoscopic approach whereby the initial cost of the robotic platform can be upwards of $1.4 million.[91,93]

SUMMARY

Laparoscopic prostatectomy allows for the safe and effective treatment of prostate cancer. Although it can be a challenging procedure early in the learning curve, continued experience can translate to progressive improvement in perioperative outcomes. Functional outcomes seem to be similar between laparoscopic and open approaches. Early oncologic outcomes are promising and suggest parity with an open approach, with equivalent long-term survival outcomes anticipated but not yet reported. Importantly, as a minimally invasive approach, laparoscopic prostatectomy remains a much cheaper alternative to the robotic approach and can achieve similar costs to an open approach with optimization of operative time and economical use of surgical supplies.

REFERENCES

1. Siegel R, Ward E, Brawley O, et al. Cancer statistics, 2011: the impact of eliminating socioeconomic and racial disparities on premature cancer deaths. CA Cancer J Clin 2011;61:212–36.
2. Stamey TA, Yang N, Hay AR, et al. Prostate-specific antigen as a serum marker for adenocarcinoma of the prostate. N Engl J Med 1987;317:909–16.
3. Catalona WJ, Smith DS, Ratliff TL, et al. Measurement of prostate-specific antigen in serum as a screening test for prostate cancer. N Engl J Med 1991; 324:1156–61.
4. Shao YH, Demissie K, Shih W, et al. Contemporary risk profile of prostate cancer in the United States. J Natl Cancer Inst 2009;101:1280–3.

5. Howlader N, Noone AM, Krapcho M, et al, editors. SEER cancer statistics review, 1975-2009. Bethesda (MD): National Cancer Institute; 2011. Available at: http://seer.cancer.gov/csr/1975_2009_pops09/.

6. Bill-Axelson A, Holmberg L, Ruutu M, et al. Radical prostatectomy versus watchful waiting in early prostate cancer. N Engl J Med 2011;364:1708–17.

7. Young HH. VIII. Conservative perineal prostatectomy: the results of two years' experience and report of seventy-five cases. Ann Surg 1905;41:549–57.

8. Oelrich TM. The urethral sphincter muscle in the male. Am J Anat 1980;158: 229–46.

9. Reiner WG, Walsh PC. An anatomical approach to the surgical management of the dorsal vein and Santorini's plexus during radical retropubic surgery. J Urol 1979;121:198–200.

10. Walsh PC, Donker PJ. Impotence following radical prostatectomy: insight into etiology and prevention. J Urol 1982;128:492–7.

11. Schuessler WW, Schulam PG, Clayman RV, et al. Laparoscopic radical prostatectomy: initial short-term experience. Urology 1997;50:854–7.

12. Abbou CC, Salomon L, Hoznek A, et al. Laparoscopic radical prostatectomy: preliminary results. Urology 2000;55:630–4.

13. Guillonneau B, Vallancien G. Laparoscopic radical prostatectomy: the Montsouris technique. J Urol 2000;163:1643–9.

14. Guillonneau B, Vallancien G. Laparoscopic radical prostatectomy: the Montsouris experience. J Urol 2000;163:418–22.

15. Poulakis V, Dillenburg W, Moeckel M, et al. Laparoscopic radical prostatectomy: prospective evaluation of the learning curve. Eur Urol 2005;47:167–75.

16. Hellawell GO, Moon DA. Laparoscopic radical prostatectomy: reducing the learning curve. Urology 2008;72:1347–50.

17. Vickers AJ, Savage CJ, Hruza M, et al. The surgical learning curve for laparoscopic radical prostatectomy: a retrospective cohort study. Lancet Oncol 2009;10:475–80.

18. Eden CG, Neill MG, Louie-Johnsun MW. The first 1000 cases of laparoscopic radical prostatectomy in the UK: evidence of multiple learning curves. BJU Int 2009;103:1224–30.

19. Siqueira TM Jr, Mitre AI, Duarte RJ, et al. Transperitoneal versus extraperitoneal laparoscopic radical prostatectomy during the learning curve: does the surgical approach affect the complication rate? Int Braz J Urol 2010;36:450–7.

20. Hruza M, Weiss HO, Pini G, et al. Complications in 2200 consecutive laparoscopic radical prostatectomies: standardised evaluation and analysis of learning curves. Eur Urol 2010;58:733–41.

21. Rodriguez AR, Rachna K, Pow-Sang JM. Laparoscopic extraperitoneal radical prostatectomy: impact of the learning curve on perioperative outcomes and margin status. JSLS 2010;14:6–13.

22. Secin FP, Savage C, Abbou C, et al. The learning curve for laparoscopic radical prostatectomy: an international multicenter study. J Urol 2010;184:2291–6.

23. Fabrizio MD, Tuerk I, Schellhammer PF. Laparoscopic radical prostatectomy: decreasing the learning curve using a mentor initiated approach. J Urol 2003; 169:2063–5.

24. Ahallal Y, Shariat SF, Chade DC, et al. Pilot study of salvage laparoscopic prostatectomy for the treatment of recurrent prostate cancer. BJU Int 2011;108:724–8.

25. Liatsikos E, Bynens B, Rabenalt R, et al. Treatment of patients after failed high intensity focused ultrasound and radiotherapy for localized prostate cancer: salvage laparoscopic extraperitoneal radical prostatectomy. J Endourol 2008;22:2295–8.

26. Patel HR, Amodeo A, Joseph JV. Salvage laparoscopic surgery in advanced prostate cancer: is it possible or beneficial? Expert Rev Anticancer Ther 2008; 8:1509–13.
27. Stolzenburg JU, Bynens B, Do M, et al. Salvage laparoscopic extraperitoneal radical prostatectomy after failed high-intensity focused ultrasound and radiotherapy for localized prostate cancer. Urology 2007;70:956–60.
28. Vallancien G, Gupta R, Cathelineau X, et al. Initial results of salvage laparoscopic radical prostatectomy after radiation failure. J Urol 2003;170:1838–40.
29. Nunez-Mora C, Garcia-Mediero JM, Cabrera-Castillo PM. Radical laparoscopic salvage prostatectomy: medium-term functional and oncological results. J Endourol 2009;23:1301–5.
30. Erdogru T, Teber D, Frede T, et al. The effect of previous transperitoneal laparoscopic inguinal herniorrhaphy on transperitoneal laparoscopic radical prostatectomy. J Urol 2005;173:769–72.
31. Stolzenburg JU, Anderson C, Rabenalt R, et al. Endoscopic extraperitoneal radical prostatectomy in patients with prostate cancer and previous laparoscopic inguinal mesh placement for hernia repair. World J Urol 2005;23:295–9.
32. Hsia M, Ponsky L, Rosenblatt S, et al. Laparoscopic inguinal hernia repair complicates future pelvic oncologic surgery. Ann Surg 2004;240:922 [author reply–3].
33. Link RE. Laparoscopic radical prostatectomy in obese patients: feasible or foolhardy? Rev Urol 2005;7:53–7.
34. Eden CG, Chang CM, Gianduzzo T, et al. The impact of obesity on laparoscopic radical prostatectomy. BJU Int 2006;98:1279–82.
35. Bhayani SB, Pavlovich CP, Strup SE, et al. Laparoscopic radical prostatectomy: a multi-institutional study of conversion to open surgery. Urology 2004;63:99–102.
36. Link BA, Nelson R, Josephson DY, et al. The impact of prostate gland weight in robot assisted laparoscopic radical prostatectomy. J Urol 2008;180:928–32.
37. Levinson AW, Bagga HS, Pavlovich CP, et al. The impact of prostate size on urinary quality of life indexes following laparoscopic radical prostatectomy. J Urol 2008;179:1818–22.
38. Molloy BL. Implications for postoperative visual loss: steep Trendelenburg position and effects on intraocular pressure. AANA J 2011;79:115–21.
39. Pandey R, Garg R, Darlong V, et al. Unpredicted neurological complications after robotic laparoscopic radical cystectomy and ileal conduit formation in steep Trendelenburg position: two case reports. Acta Anaesthesiol Belg 2010; 61:163–6.
40. Rosevear HM, Lightfoot AJ, Zahs M, et al. Lessons learned from a case of calf compartment syndrome after robot-assisted laparoscopic prostatectomy. J Endourol 2010;24:1597–601.
41. Kalmar AF, Foubert L, Hendrickx JF, et al. Influence of steep Trendelenburg position and CO(2) pneumoperitoneum on cardiovascular, cerebrovascular, and respiratory homeostasis during robotic prostatectomy. Br J Anaesth 2010; 104:433–9.
42. Rodriguez AR, Kapoor R, Pow-Sang JM. Laparoscopic extraperitoneal radical prostatectomy in complex surgical cases. J Urol 2007;177:1765–70.
43. Porpiglia F, Terrone C, Tarabuzzi R, et al. Transperitoneal versus extraperitoneal laparoscopic radical prostatectomy: experience of a single center. Urology 2006;68:376–80.

44. Cathelineau X, Cahill D, Widmer H, et al. Transperitoneal or extraperitoneal approach for laparoscopic radical prostatectomy: a false debate over a real challenge. J Urol 2004;171:714–6.
45. Hoznek A, Antiphon P, Borkowski T, et al. Assessment of surgical technique and perioperative morbidity associated with extraperitoneal versus transperitoneal laparoscopic radical prostatectomy. Urology 2003;61:617–22.
46. Eden CG, King D, Kooiman GG, et al. Transperitoneal or extraperitoneal laparoscopic radical prostatectomy: does the approach matter? J Urol 2004;172: 2218–23.
47. Erdogru T, Teber D, Frede T, et al. Comparison of transperitoneal and extraperitoneal laparoscopic radical prostatectomy using match-pair analysis. Eur Urol 2004;46:312–9 [discussion: 20].
48. Atug F, Castle EP, Woods M, et al. Transperitoneal versus extraperitoneal robotic-assisted radical prostatectomy: is one better than the other? Urology 2006;68:1077–81.
49. Landman J, Venkatesh R, Vanlangendonck R, et al. Application of a fixed retractor system to facilitate laparoscopic radical prostatectomy. J Urol 2004; 171:783–5.
50. Bhayani SB, Andriole GL. Three-dimensional (3D) vision: does it improve laparoscopic skills? An assessment of a 3D head-mounted visualization system. Rev Urol 2005;7:211–4.
51. Thurairaja R, Studer UE, Burkhard FC. Indications, extent, and benefits of pelvic lymph node dissection for patients with bladder and prostate cancer. Oncologist 2009;14:40–51.
52. Clarebrough EE, Challacombe BJ, Briggs C, et al. Cadaveric analysis of periprostatic nerve distribution: an anatomical basis for high anterior release during radical prostatectomy? J Urol 2011;185:1519–25.
53. Van Velthoven RF, Ahlering TE, Peltier A, et al. Technique for laparoscopic running urethrovesical anastomosis: the single knot method. Urology 2003;61: 699–702.
54. Bhayani SB, Pavlovich CP, Hsu TS, et al. Prospective comparison of short-term convalescence: laparoscopic radical prostatectomy versus open radical retropubic prostatectomy. Urology 2003;61:612–6.
55. Egawa S, Kuruma H, Suyama K, et al. Delayed recovery of urinary continence after laparoscopic radical prostatectomy. Int J Urol 2003;10:207–12.
56. Roumeguere T, Bollens R, Vanden Bossche M, et al. Radical prostatectomy: a prospective comparison of oncological and functional results between open and laparoscopic approaches. World J Urol 2003;20:360–6.
57. Brown JA, Garlitz C, Gomella LG, et al. Perioperative morbidity of laparoscopic radical prostatectomy compared with open radical retropubic prostatectomy. Urol Oncol 2004;22:102–6.
58. Guazzoni G, Cestari A, Naspro R, et al. Intra- and peri-operative outcomes comparing radical retropubic and laparoscopic radical prostatectomy: results from a prospective, randomised, single-surgeon study. Eur Urol 2006;50: 98–104.
59. Jurczok A, Zacharias M, Wagner S, et al. Prospective non-randomized evaluation of four mediators of the systemic response after extraperitoneal laparoscopic and open retropubic radical prostatectomy. BJU Int 2007;99: 1461–6.
60. Poulakis V, Witzsch U, de Vries R, et al. Laparoscopic radical prostatectomy in men older than 70 years of age with localized prostate cancer: comparison of

morbidity, reconvalescence, and short-term clinical outcomes between younger and older men. Eur Urol 2007;51:1341–8 [discussion: 9].

61. Touijer K, Eastham JA, Secin FP, et al. Comprehensive prospective comparative analysis of outcomes between open and laparoscopic radical prostatectomy conducted in 2003 to 2005. J Urol 2008;179:1811–7 [discussion: 7].

62. Anastasiadis AG, Salomon L, Katz R, et al. Radical retropubic versus laparoscopic prostatectomy: a prospective comparison of functional outcome. Urology 2003;62:292–7.

63. Holzbeierlein JM, Smith JA. Radical prostatectomy and collaborative care pathways. Semin Urol Oncol 2000;18:60–5.

64. Yu HY, Hevelone ND, Lipsitz SR, et al. Use, costs and comparative effectiveness of robotic assisted, laparoscopic and open urological surgery. J Urol 2012; 187(4):1392–8.

65. Ficarra V, Novara G, Artibani W, et al. Retropubic, laparoscopic, and robot-assisted radical prostatectomy: a systematic review and cumulative analysis of comparative studies. Eur Urol 2009;55:1037–63.

66. Joseph JV, Vicente I, Madeb R, et al. Robot-assisted vs pure laparoscopic radical prostatectomy: are there any differences? BJU Int 2005;96:39–42.

67. Menon M, Shrivastava A, Tewari A, et al. Laparoscopic and robot assisted radical prostatectomy: establishment of a structured program and preliminary analysis of outcomes. J Urol 2002;168:945–9.

68. Rozet F, Jaffe J, Braud G, et al. A direct comparison of robotic assisted versus pure laparoscopic radical prostatectomy: a single institution experience. J Urol 2007;178:478–82.

69. Rassweiler J, Schulze M, Teber D, et al. Laparoscopic radical prostatectomy with the Heilbronn technique: oncological results in the first 500 patients. J Urol 2005;173:761–4.

70. Tai HC, Lai MK, Huang CY, et al. Oncologic outcomes of Asian men with clinically localized prostate cancer after extraperitoneal laparoscopic radical prostatectomy: a single-institution experience. Prostate Cancer 2011;2011:748616.

71. Paul A, Ploussard G, Nicolaiew N, et al. Oncologic outcome after extraperitoneal laparoscopic radical prostatectomy: midterm follow-up of 1115 procedures. Eur Urol 2010;57:267–72.

72. Rassweiler J, Stolzenburg J, Sulser T, et al. Laparoscopic radical prostatectomy–the experience of the German Laparoscopic Working Group. Eur Urol 2006;49:113–9.

73. Roehl KA, Han M, Ramos CG, et al. Cancer progression and survival rates following anatomical radical retropubic prostatectomy in 3,478 consecutive patients: long-term results. J Urol 2004;172:910–4.

74. Han M, Partin AW, Pound CR, et al. Long-term biochemical disease-free and cancer-specific survival following anatomic radical retropubic prostatectomy. The 15-year Johns Hopkins experience. Urol Clin North Am 2001;28:555–65.

75. Catalona WJ, Smith DS. 5-year tumor recurrence rates after anatomical radical retropubic prostatectomy for prostate cancer. J Urol 1994;152:1837–42.

76. Zincke H, Bergstralh EJ, Blute ML, et al. Radical prostatectomy for clinically localized prostate cancer: long-term results of 1,143 patients from a single institution. J Clin Oncol 1994;12:2254–63.

77. Litwin MS, Hays RD, Fink A, et al. Quality-of-life outcomes in men treated for localized prostate cancer. JAMA 1995;273:129–35.

78. Sanda MG, Dunn RL, Michalski J, et al. Quality of life and satisfaction with outcome among prostate-cancer survivors. N Engl J Med 2008;358:1250–61.

79. Rassweiler J, Seemann O, Schulze M, et al. Laparoscopic versus open radical prostatectomy: a comparative study at a single institution. J Urol 2003;169: 1689–93.

80. Romero-Otero J, Touijer K, Guillonneau B. Laparoscopic radical prostatectomy: contemporary comparison with open surgery. Urol Oncol 2007;25:499–504.

81. Guillonneau B, Cathelineau X, Doublet JD, et al. Laparoscopic radical prostatectomy: assessment after 550 procedures. Crit Rev Oncol Hematol 2002;43: 123–33.

82. Rozet F, Galiano M, Cathelineau X, et al. Extraperitoneal laparoscopic radical prostatectomy: a prospective evaluation of 600 cases. J Urol 2005;174:908–11.

83. Stolzenburg JU, Rabenalt R, Do M, et al. Endoscopic extraperitoneal radical prostatectomy: oncological and functional results after 700 procedures. J Urol 2005;174:1271–5 [discussion: 5].

84. Curto F, Benijts J, Pansadoro A, et al. Nerve sparing laparoscopic radical prostatectomy: our technique. Eur Urol 2006;49:344–52.

85. Salomon L, Anastasiadis AG, Katz R, et al. Urinary continence and erectile function: a prospective evaluation of functional results after radical laparoscopic prostatectomy. Eur Urol 2002;42:338–43.

86. Hoznek A, Salomon L, Olsson LE, et al. Laparoscopic radical prostatectomy. The Creteil experience. Eur Urol 2001;40:38–45.

87. Link RE, Su LM, Sullivan W, et al. Health related quality of life before and after laparoscopic radical prostatectomy. J Urol 2005;173:175–9 [discussion: 9].

88. Rassweiler J, Schulze M, Teber D, et al. Laparoscopic radical prostatectomy: functional and oncological outcomes. Curr Opin Urol 2004;14:75–82.

89. Turk I, Deger S, Winkelmann B, et al. Laparoscopic radical prostatectomy. Technical aspects and experience with 125 cases. Eur Urol 2001;40:46–52 [discussion: 3].

90. Link RE, Su LM, Bhayani SB, et al. Making ends meet: a cost comparison of laparoscopic and open radical retropubic prostatectomy. J Urol 2004;172: 269–74.

91. Lotan Y, Cadeddu JA, Gettman MT. The new economics of radical prostatectomy: cost comparison of open, laparoscopic and robot assisted techniques. J Urol 2004;172:1431–5.

92. Anderson JK, Murdock A, Cadeddu JA, et al. Cost comparison of laparoscopic versus radical retropubic prostatectomy. Urology 2005;66:557–60.

93. Bolenz C, Gupta A, Hotze T, et al. Cost comparison of robotic, laparoscopic, and open radical prostatectomy for prostate cancer. Eur Urol 2010;57:453–8.

94. Lein M, Stibane I, Mansour R, et al. Complications, urinary continence, and oncologic outcome of 1000 laparoscopic transperitoneal radical prostatectomies-experience at the Charite Hospital Berlin, Campus Mitte. Eur Urol 2006;50:1278–82 [discussion: 83–4].

95. Eden CG, Cahill D, Vass JA, et al. Laparoscopic radical prostatectomy: the initial UK series. BJU Int 2002;90:876–82.

96. Ferguson GG, Humphrey PA, Andriole GL. Margin status of men undergoing extraperitoneal, extrafascial laparoscopic radical prostatectomy (abstract 1771). In: AUA annual meeting program abstracts. Orlando (FL): J Urol. 2008. p. 179:607.

97. Cohen MS, Triaca V, Silverman ML, et al. Progression of laparoscopic radical prostatectomy: improved outcomes with the extraperitoneal approach and a running anastomosis. J Endourol 2006;20:574–9.

98. Goeman L, Salomon L, La De Taille A, et al. Long-term functional and oncological results after retroperitoneal laparoscopic prostatectomy according to a prospective evaluation of 550 patients. World J Urol 2006;24:281–8.

99. Stolzenburg JU, Rabenalt R, Do M, et al. Endoscopic extraperitoneal radical prostatectomy: the University of Leipzig experience of 2000 cases. J Endourol 2008;22:2319–25.
100. Zincke H, Oesterling JE, Blute ML, et al. Long-term (15 years) results after radical prostatectomy for clinically localized (stage T2c or lower) prostate cancer. J Urol 1994;152:1850–7.
101. Lepor H, Nieder AM, Ferrandino MN. Intraoperative and postoperative complications of radical retropubic prostatectomy in a consecutive series of 1,000 cases. J Urol 2001;166:1729–33.
102. Guillonneau B, el-Fettouh H, Baumert H, et al. Laparoscopic radical prostatectomy: oncological evaluation after 1,000 cases a Montsouris Institute. J Urol 2003;169:1261–6.
103. Pavlovich CP, Trock BJ, Sulman A. 3-year actuarial biochemical recurrence-free survival following laparoscopic radical prostatectomy: experience from a tertiary referral center in the United States. J Urol 2008;179:917–21 [discussion: 21–2].

Lap Colectomy and Robotics for Colon Cancer

Eduardo Parra-Davila, MD[a],*, Sonia Ramamoorthy, MD[b]

KEYWORDS

• Robotic • Colon cancer • Minimal invasive colectomy

KEY POINTS

• Early data show favorable perioperative outcomes for robotic-assisted colectomy for colon cancer.
• Increasingly, surgeons are applying minimally invasive techniques to colon cancer surgery; robotics may represent the next evolution of this trend.
• Disadvantages of robotics include cost, learning curve, and length of surgery; however, these disadvantages must be balanced with the reported advantages of successful mesocolic dissection, surgeon preference, and enhanced surgeon capabilities.
• Long-term prospective studies are needed to determine if robotic colectomy for colon cancer surgery offers similar or better outcomes when compared with traditional approaches.

INTRODUCTION

The original application of the current robotic platform was in cardiac surgery. The robot offered increased surgeon dexterity in a small field with the added advantage of a minimally invasive approach. The creation of the robotic surgery system drastically changed the surgical management in different specialties since 2001 when the first robotic prostatectomy was performed in Germany.[1] Many specialties were impacted by robotic technology, including urology, gynecology, and head and neck surgery. Over time, clinical data from these series matured enough to demonstrate safety, efficiency, reproducibility, and oncologic and functional outcomes comparable with its open and laparoscopic counterparts.[2–4] This awareness has brought the robot to its current and most widely used application, the robotic prostatectomy. During the adoption phase of robotics into urology, minimally invasive surgical techniques were being studied in colorectal cancer surgery.

The results of the Clinical Outcomes of Surgical Therapy (COST) trial in 2004 concluded that laparoscopic approaches to colon cancer could be performed without

[a] Florida Hospital Celebration Health Campus, Celebration Colorectal, 410 Celebration Place, Suite 401, Celebration, FL 34747, USA; [b] Division of Colon and Rectal Surgery, University of California San Diego Health System, 855 Health Sciences Drive La Jolla, San Diego, CA 92093-0987, USA
* Corresponding author.
E-mail address: Eduardo.parradavila.md@flhosp.org

Surg Oncol Clin N Am 22 (2013) 143–151
http://dx.doi.org/10.1016/j.soc.2012.08.007
1055-3207/13/$ – see front matter © 2013 Published by Elsevier Inc.

the compromise of oncologic or quality-of-life outcomes.[5] Worldwide, more than 1 million people develop colorectal cancer annually (with approximately 608 000 deaths), accounting for 8% of all cancer deaths, making it the fourth cause of death from all cancers.[6] Minimally invasive approaches are rapidly gaining acceptance among colorectal and general surgeons. Recent data have shown that between 10% and 30% of colon surgeries are currently being performed using laparoscopic techniques in the United States.[7] Barriers to the widespread adoption of laparoscopy include education and training, steep learning curve, personal experience, access to trained assistants, financial reimbursement, length of surgery, and patient availability.[7] Surprisingly, despite these challenges, robotic approaches for the management of colon cancer are slowly gaining momentum, which brings the discussion to the topic of this article: the application of robotics to colon cancer surgery. To date, the most significant application of robotics in colorectal surgery is for rectal cancer surgery; however, increasingly surgeons are applying this technology to intra-abdominal procedures, such as colectomy. In this article, the authors review the advantages and disadvantages of robotic-assisted colectomy and the techniques, early outcomes, and future directions.

CURRENT INDICATIONS

Robotic surgery was introduced to colorectal surgery to overcome the challenges of a minimally invasive dissection in the narrow deep pelvis. Surgeons were curious to see if the system could overcome the pitfalls of laparoscopic surgery with better oncologic and functional outcomes. In the past 5 years, there have been increasing numbers of early outcome studies published on robotic-assisted rectal cancer surgery demonstrating feasibility and safety and without deterioration in oncologic and functional outcomes.[8,9] Although most of the studies of robotic-assisted colorectal surgery report on early experience and lack the power of larger series, there are 2 multicenter, prospective, cooperative clinical trials underway to compare robotic assisted rectal cancer surgery with laparoscopic (robotic versus laparoscopic resection for rectal cancer [ROLLAR]) and open techniques (American College of Surgeons Oncology Group 6051).[10,11] These studies have stimulated increased interest in robotic colorectal surgery, which has lead to interest in applying these very same techniques to colectomy.

ADVANTAGES OF ROBOTIC SURGERY

The reported advantages of robotic surgery include all the advantages of minimally invasive surgery plus the following:

- Three-dimensional (3D) HD vision: This vision is better than 2-dimensional high definition (HD), giving the surgeons the depth perception without the learning curve of adapting to it, as is the case with laparoscopy.
- Visual magnification: The robot is capable of magnifying images 10 to 15 times normal, which is more than what is seen with standard laparoscopy and much more than the naked eye. This magnification allows the surgeon to be more selective about the dissection of critical structures by fractions of a millimeter.
- Motion scaling: In standard laparoscopy, the distance of the tissue structure from the port site on the abdomen causes amplification of motion at the instrument tip. A small motion outside the body causes a relatively large motion on the inside. This motion can frustrate attempts to target tissues. With the surgical robot, motions are filtered and deamplified up to a scale of 5 to 1. In other words, the surgeon would have to move the manipulators up to 5 in to cause movement of only an inch on the inside of the body. This motion scaling eliminates natural

hand tremor entirely, allows the surgeon to target tissues with much greater ease, and gives the surgeon a certain finesse that surpasses human capabilities in both the open and standard laparoscopic realms.

- Ergonomics: In standard laparoscopy, the surgeon must stand, sometimes in rather awkward positions, for several hours. This position can cause fatigue and long-term disability. With the surgical robot, however, the surgeon is seated comfortably at a console. The hands are positioned in a natural forward position, and the forearms are given a rest to lean on. This configuration relieves much stress on the operating surgeon and that often translates to a better quality surgery for patients.
- Endowrist technology (Intuitive Surgical, Inc, Sunnyvale, CA): Standard laparoscopy uses fixed instrument tips. The surgical robot, however, has instrument tips that rotate and angulate in multiple different directions. This ability allows for imitation of normal wrist and elbow motions. This technology is capable of spinning 2 full revolutions, whereas the human hand can only turn about 270°.
- Telementoring and telesurgery: The future of surgery is to teach and operate from the distance, which will allow us to perform surgery at remote areas of the world where minimally invasive surgery is not available.

The combination of these various elements gives the surgeon a sense of total control over the operation. Together, these reported advantages can translate into the following clinical advantages: facilitating sphincter preservation in low rectal tumors, ease of intracorporeal suturing, adoption of natural orifice surgery, and the use of alternate extraction sites that may decrease the rate of abdominal wall hernias and decrease pain in the patients.

DISADVANTAGES OF ROBOTIC SURGERY

Despite the multiple advantages of robotic surgery, few can deny that there are educational, fiscal, and access barriers that exist to the adoption of this technology.

- Time: Most robotic series report longer operative times when compared with multiport laparoscopy. Although this variable can be altered with the surgeon's expertise, the most experienced surgeons are equally as efficient on both techniques. In a longer surgery, patient are under anesthesia for longer and it costs more to staff the procedure.[8,12]
- Cost: At this early stage in the technology, robotic systems are very expensive. Several early outcome studies have demonstrated increased costs with robotics when compared with open and laparoscopic techniques.[12,13] Improvements in technology and more competition in the market will likely reduce costs in the future. However, current modifications, service contracts, and technological advances have driven costs up, not down, and created an ever-increasing fiscal burden on hospitals and academic institutions. Another issue with costs is the problem with upgrading the systems as they improve. Only when these systems gain more widespread multidisciplinary use, will the costs become more justified. Currently, there are no specific reimbursements for robotic-assisted colorectal procedures.
- Difficulty approaching multi-quadrant procedures: The arms of the robot come from a center column and have a certain degree of motion related to where this column is placed. Most of the time, the column is placed in line with the area of disease or target organ. In colorectal cases involving patients with a larger body mass index, there is the need for double-docking techniques to be able to avoid collisions of the robotic arms, specifically in low anterior resection when mobilization of the splenic flexure is needed.

- Loss of tactile or haptic sensation: This problem was one of the criticisms of laparoscopic surgery; however, this problem is further accentuated with robotics. Surgeons with experience are able to compensate by using "visual haptics" which refers to the ability to adjust tissue pressure based on visual cues.
- Learning curve: There is a learning curve associated with robotic technology. Frustrations with equipment setup and port placement can be alleviated with experienced bedside assistants. Previous investigators have reported that surgeons skilled in laparoscopic colorectal surgery progress through 3 phases when applying robotic techniques.[14] Using cumulative sum (CUSUM) analysis, the investigators noted that the initial phase consisted of 15 cases whereby the initial learning curve took place. Phase 2 represented a plateau phase whereby surgeons were primarily becoming more accustomed to the robotic console and gaining competence. Finally, phase 3 represented the mastery phase after 25 total cases and consisted of the adequate skills needed to perform routine cases skillfully and embark on more challenging cases.

When reviewing the disadvantages of robotic surgery, it is clear that the major obstacle to widespread use is the longer operative times (learning curve) and increased costs. It is important, however, to recognize that, for both the learning curve and the operative duration, having consistent robotic teams familiar with the robot, its setup, potential malfunctions, and operative approaches can have a significant impact on reducing the operative time and reducing surgeon frustration. This familiarity can impact patient outcomes and total costs. Advocates of robotic surgery argue that the cost of the system can be balanced when examining cost savings and the return on investment more broadly; high-volume robotic centers offset costs by increasing use, reducing the length of stay, and having less morbidity and early return to work/quality of life. This situation seems to be the case in robotic-assisted prostatectomy when compared with open prostatectomy; however, these reported cost savings have not been demonstrated in colorectal surgery to date.[15]

EARLY OUTCOMES FOR ROBOTIC-ASSISTED COLECTOMY

Early outcome data suggest that robotic-assisted colectomy is both safe and feasible.[16–18] Most will agree that the advantages that are pertinent to the rectum during the pelvic dissection could also apply to colectomy. Most of the series published are nonrandomized or comparative studies that preclude definitive conclusions; but this early data show equivalent clinical and oncologic short-term outcomes, except for longer operating times and a lower conversion rate when compared with laparoscopic surgery (**Table 1**). In a review of robotic colorectal cases to date, Antoniou and colleagues[23] concluded that right colectomies seem to benefit from a robotic approach, with a reduction in the conversion rate and lower complication rates when compared with laparoscopy. There are technical limits in conventional laparoscopic surgery that are more pronounced in obese patients or in cases that require increased technical skill because of the complexity of the disease, such as a T4 colon cancer. Instrumentation specific to robotics can make possible cases that were once thought to be contraindications to minimally invasive surgery.

ONCOLOGIC CONSIDERATIONS

The adequacy of the mesocolic resection for colon cancer is undoubtedly one of the most important outcomes when discussing minimally invasive approaches to colon cancer surgery. In a study of more than 399 colectomy cases, West and colleagues[24]

Table 1			
Early outcomes for robotic-assisted colectomy			
Author, Year	Number of Cases	Type (Number of Cases)	Outcome (Robot vs Laparoscopic)
Delaney et al,[17] 2003	6	Right (2), sigmoid (3), rectopexy (1)	Time: 165 min vs 108 min Complications: LOS, EBL: NS
Anvari et al,[19] 2004	10	Right (5), left (2), LAR (2), subtotal (1)	Time: 155.3 min vs 94.4 min Complications: LOS, EBL: NS
D'Annibale et al,[20] 2004	53	Right (10), left (28), LAR (10), APR (1), total colectomy (2), Hartmann (1), rectopexy (1)	Time: 240 min vs 222 min Complications: LOS, EBL: NS
Spinoglio et al,[21] 2008	50	Right (18), left (10), LAR (19), APR (1), transverse colectomy (1), total colectomy (1)	Time: 383 min vs 266 min Complications: LOS: NS
Rawlings et al,[16] 2006	30	Right (17), sigmoid (13)	Right hemicolectomy: Time: 218.9 min vs 169.2 min Complications: LOS, EBL: NS
deSouza et al,[13] 2010	40	Right (40)	Time: 158.9 min vs 118.0 min Complications: LOS, EBL: NS
Deutsch et al,[22] 2012	171	Right (65), left (106)	Time: 140 min vs 135 min for right colectomy; mean 168 min vs 203 min for left colectomy Complications: LOS, EBL: NS

Abbreviations: APR, abdominal-perineal resection; EBL, estimated blood loss; LAR, low anterior resection; LOS, length of stay; NS, no statistical difference.

describe marked pathologic variation in the proportion of each plane of surgery: muscularis propria in 95 out of 399 (24%) specimens, intramesocolic in 177 out of 399 (44%) specimens, and mesocolic in 127 out of 399 (32%) specimens. These findings translated into a 15% (95% confidence interval) overall survival advantage at 5 years with mesocolic plane surgery compared with surgery in the muscularis propria plane and was significant in patients with stage III cancers. In a study by Chang and colleagues,[25] the number of lymph nodes harvested was positively correlated with survival in stage I and II colon cancer. In the COST trial, it was shown that a laparoscopic approach is as at least as adequate as an open approach with regard to margins and lymph node harvest.[7] Similarly, early studies in robotic-assisted surgery for colon cancer have shown similar oncologic outcomes to open and laparoscopic surgery (**Table 2**). In a direct comparison of robotic surgery with open surgery colon cancer outcomes, Luca and colleagues[29] found longer operative times with the robotic arm; but they found reduced blood loss, longer specimen length, and increased nodes when compared with case-matched open resection. The investigators suggest that enhanced visualization and endowrist movements provide the necessary technical advantages to perform an appropriate mesocolic resection. Future randomized trials with an emphasis on the pathologic grading of specimen are needed to confirm if robotic-assisted surgery is indeed a superior tool for performing minimally invasive colon cancer surgery.

The safety and feasibility of robotic assistance in right hemicolectomy has been demonstrated in several published reports (see **Table 2**). However, no report was able to demonstrate an objective advantage for the robot over conventional multiport laparoscopy. Moreover, the use of the robot is associated with a longer operating

Table 2
Robotic-assisted colectomy for colon cancer

Author, Year	Number of Cases	Type (Number of Cases)	Outcome (Robot vs Laparoscopic)
D'Annibale et al,[20] 2004	53	Right (10), left (28), LAR (10), APR (1), total colectomy (2)	Lymph nodes: 16 vs 19 (ns) Margin: neg
Spinoglio et al,[21] 2008	50	Right (18), left (10), LAR (19), APR (1), transverse colectomy (1), total colectomy (1)	Lymph nodes: 22.03 vs 22.85 Margin: neg
deSouza,[26] 2010	40	Right (42)	Lymph nodes: 19 Margins: neg
Deutsch et al,[22] 2012	171	Right (65), left (106)	Lymph nodes: 21.1 vs 18.7 (right) 10 vs 30 (left) Margins: neg
Buchs et al,[27] 2012	3	Right (3)	Lymph nodes: 18 Margins: neg
Shin JY,[28] 2012	30	Right (12), left (19)	Lymph nodes: 18 vs 15 Margins: neg

Abbreviations: APR, abdomino-perineal resection; LAR, low anterior resection.

time and a higher cost, questioning the role of the robot in this procedure when multi-port laparoscopy has been shown to be safe, oncologically sound, and demonstrated to cost less and have reduced operating room times when compared with robotics. A right hemicolectomy, on the other hand, is a relatively less challenging procedure and can be performed with just 2 robotic instrument arms. Additionally, conversion to either the open or laparoscopic approach can easily be achieved should the need arise. The procedure is, therefore, an excellent learning tool and is ideally suited to begin clinical experience with the robot. Once the basic techniques of robotic surgery have been acquired, more advanced procedures can be attempted.

FUTURE DIRECTIONS
Intracorporeal Anastomosis

Increasingly, surgeons are gaining interest in performing intracorporeal hand-sewn anastomosis. The advantages of this approach are unproven but reported to be reduced length of extraction incision; reduced risk of wound complications; and the ability to facilitate alternate extractions sites, such as a natural orifice extraction (trans-vaginal) or an extraction through a Pfannenstiel incision, which is associated with fewer complications and a significantly lower hernia rate. This procedure would be significantly more technically challenging with conventional laparoscopy, but it is made easier with the 3D imaging and endowrist movement of the robot. The optimal technique for a robotic hand-sewn intracorporeal colon anastomosis is still being developed, and the results on the complications and leak rates associated with this technique are still awaited.

Single-Incision Surgery

Single-incision laparoscopic colon surgery is a recent concept that is being exten-sively investigated. The crossing of laparoscopic instruments in this technique places the instrument controlled by the surgeon's right hand on the left side of the screen and vice versa. This technique can be quite challenging and is considered an advanced laparoscopic technique that is associated with a steep learning curve. Still, single-incision colectomy is gaining wide acceptance as an alternate to multi-port laparoscopy in ideal patients. Single-incision technology was recently introduced to the robotic platform; however, before this it could be preformed on a standard platform by switching masters, and control of the instrument on one side of the visual field could be assigned to the ipsilateral hand, although the instruments were crossed. This feature of the da Vinci robot (Intuitive Surgical, Sunnyvale, CA) has significant potential in single-incision surgery because it can be applied to abdominal, endoluminal, and transanal procedures (Larach). The feasibility of a robot-assisted single-incision right hemicolectomy is currently being evaluated, and an initial report on the early experience with this technique has recently been published.[10]

Fluorescein dye laser imaging is the latest advance in robotic surgery that assists the surgeon with visualization of the vascular structures. This advance may be seen as the earliest form of image-guided surgery. To date, this technology is thought to assist with better identification of vascular structures; in the future, it could be used to identify sentinel nodes and assess anastomotic perfusion and neurovascular structures to limit postoperative disability.

SUMMARY

In conclusion, robotic surgery is rapidly gaining wide acceptance as an alternative platform for minimally invasive surgery. The current application for robotics in colorectal surgery is in rectal cancer surgery. However, robotic surgery for colon cancer is increasing; in the future, clinical trials and long-term outcomes will ultimately determine its future.

REFERENCES

1. Kramer BJ. Robotically – assisted laparoscopic radical prostatectomy. BJU Int 2001;87:408–10.
2. Patel VR, Palmer KJ, Coughlin G, et al. Robot assisted laparoscopic radical prostatectomy: perioperative outcomes of 1500 cases. J Endourol 2008;22: 2299–305.
3. Zora KC, Gofrit ON, Steinberg GP, et al. Planned nerve preservation to reduce positive surgical margins during robot-assisted laparoscopic radical prostatectomy. J Endourol 2008;22:1303–9.
4. Badani KK, Kaul S, MEnon M. Evolution of robotic radical prostatectomy: assessment after 2766 procedures. Cancer 2007;110:1951–8.
5. The Clinical Outcomes of Surgical Therapy Study Group. A comparison of laparoscopically assisted and open colectomy for colon cancer. N Engl J Med 2004; 350:2050–9.
6. World Health Statistics Annual: WHO Databank. Available at: http-dep-arc.fr/. Accessed July 19, 2010.
7. Steele SR, Stein SL, Bordeianou LG, et al, American Society of Colon and Rectal Surgeons' Young Surgeons Committee. The impact of practice environment on laparoscopic colectomy utilization following colorectal residency, 2012: a survey of the ASCRS Young Surgeons. Colorectal Dis 2012;14(3):374–81.
8. Baik SH, Kwon HY, Kim JS, et al. Robotic versus laparoscopic low anterior resection of rectal cancer: short-term outcome of a prospective comparative study. Ann Surg Oncol 2009;16(6):1480–7.

9. Patriti A, Ceacrelli G, Bartoli A, et al. Short and medium term outcome of robotic assisted and traditional laparoscopic rectal resection. JSLS 2009;13: 176–83.

10. Collinson FJ, Jayne DG, Pigazzi A, et al. An international, multicentre, prospective, randomised, controlled, unblinded, parallel-group trial of robotic-assisted versus standard laparoscopic surgery for the curative treatment of rectal cancer. Int J Colorectal Dis 2012;27(2):233–41.

11. Baik SH, Gincherman M, Mutch MG, et al. Laparoscopic vs. open resection for patients with rectal cancer: comparison of perioperative outcomes and long-term survival. Dis Colon Rectum 2011;54(1):6–14.

12. Heemskerk J, de Hoog DE, van Gemert WG, et al. Robot-assisted vs. conventional laparoscopic rectopexy for rectal prolapse: a comparative study on costs and time. Dis Colon Rectum 2007;50(11):1825–30.

13. deSouza AL, Prasad LM, Park JJ, et al. Robotic assistance in right hemicolectomy: is there a role? Dis Colon Rectum 2010;53(7):1000–6.

14. Bokhari MB, Patel CB, Ramos-Valadez DI, et al. Learning curve for robotic-assisted laparoscopic colorectal surgery. Surg Endosc 2011;25(3):855–60.

15. Anderson JE, Chang DC, Parsons JK, et al. The first national examination of outcomes and trends in robotic surgery in the United States. J Am Coll Surg 2012;215:107–14.

16. Rawlings AL, Woodland JH, Crawford DL. Telerobotic surgery for right and sigmoid colectomies: 30 consecutive cases. Surg Endosc 2006;20(11):1713–8.

17. Delaney CP, Lynch AC, Senagore AJ, et al. Comparison of robotically performed and traditional laparoscopic colorectal surgery. Dis Colon Rectum 2003;46(12): 1633–9.

18. Braumann C, Jacobi CA, Menenakos C, et al. Computer-assisted laparoscopic colon resection with the da Vinci system: our first experiences. Dis Colon Rectum 2005;48(9):1820–7.

19. Anvari M, Birch DW, Bamehriz F, et al. Robotic-assisted laparoscopic colorectal surgery. Surg Laparosc Endosc Percutan Tech 2004;14(6):311–5.

20. D'Annibale A, Morpurgo E, Fiscon V, et al. Robotic and laparoscopic surgery for treatment of colorectal diseases. Dis Colon Rectum 2004;47(12):2162–8.

21. Spinoglio G, Summa M, Priora F, et al. Robotic colorectal surgery: first 50 cases experience. Dis Colon Rectum 2008;51(11):1627–32.

22. Deutsch GB, Sathyanarayana SA, Gunabushanam V, et al. Robotic vs. laparoscopic colorectal surgery: an institutional experience. Surg Endosc 2012;26(4): 956–63.

23. Antoniou SA, Antoniou GA, Koch OO, et al. Robot-assisted laparoscopic surgery of the colon and rectum [review]. Surg Endosc 2012;26(1):1–11.

24. West NP, Morris EJ, Rotimi O, et al. Pathology grading of colon cancer surgical resection and its association with survival: a retrospective observational study. Lancet Oncol 2008;9(9):857–65.

25. Chang GJ, Rodriguez-Bigas MA, Skibber JM, et al. Lymph node evaluation and survival after curative resection of colon cancer: systematic review. J Natl Cancer Inst 2007;99(6):433–41.

26. Zimmern A, Prasad L, deSouza A, et al. Robotic colon and rectal surgery: a series of 131 cases. World J Surg 2010;34:1954–8.

27. Buchs N, Pugin F, Bucher P, et al. Totally robotic right colectomy: preliminary case series and an overview of the literature. Int J Med Robot 2011. [Epub ahead of print].

28. Shin JY. Comparison of short term oncologic outcomes between a robotic colectomy and a laparoscopic colectomy during early experience. J Korean Soc Coloproctol 2012;28(1):19–26.
29. Luca F, Ghezzi TL, Valvo M, et al. Surgical and pathological outcomes after right hemicolectomy: case-matched study comparing robotic and open surgery. Int J Med Robot 2011. [Epub ahead of print]. http://dx.doi.org/10.1002/rcs.398.

Index

Note: Page numbers of article titles are in **boldface** type.

Moving?

Make sure your subscription moves with you!

To notify us of your new address, find your **Clinics Account Number** (located on your mailing label above your name), and contact customer service at:

Email: journalscustomerservice-usa@elsevier.com

800-654-2452 (subscribers in the U.S. & Canada)
314-447-8871 (subscribers outside of the U.S. & Canada)

Fax number: 314-447-8029

Elsevier Health Sciences Division
Subscription Customer Service
3251 Riverport Lane
Maryland Heights, MO 63043

*To ensure uninterrupted delivery of your subscription, please notify us at least 4 weeks in advance of move.

Printed and bound by CPI Group (UK) Ltd, Croydon, CR0 4YY

03/10/2024

01040440-0017